The Healing Power of Herbs

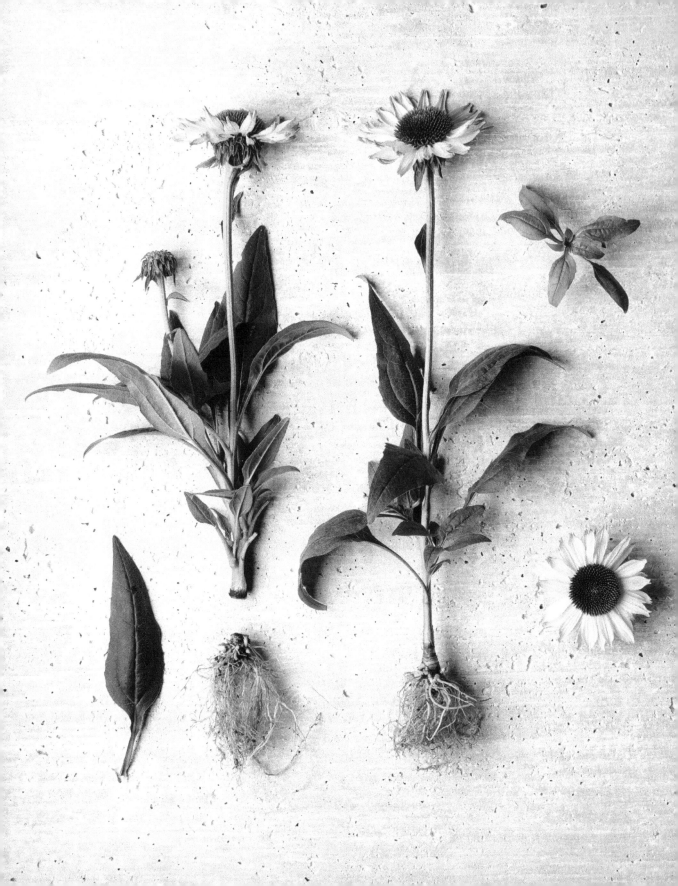

the HEALING POWER of HERBS

Medicinal Herbs for Common Ailments

Tina Sams

PHOTOGRAPHY BY
Marija Vidal

ALTHEA
PRESS

For general information on our other products and services or to obtain technical support, please contact our Customer Care Department within the U.S. at (866) 744-2665, or outside the U.S. at (510) 253-0500.

Althea Press publishes its books in a variety of electronic and print formats. Some content that appears in print may not be available in electronic books, and vice versa.

Interior and Cover Designer: Emma Hall
Photo Art Director / Art Manager: Karen Beard
Editor: Vanessa Ta
Production Editor: Erum Khan
Photography © 2018 Marija Vidal. Food styling by Cregg Green.
Illustration © Foxyliam/Shutterstock.
Author photo © 2018 Maryanne Schwartz.

ISBN Print 978-1-64152-239-7 | eBook 978-1-64152-240-3

To chamomile, elder, holy basil, and mimosa—my favorite teachers.
To Molly and Maryanne for keeping me laughing.

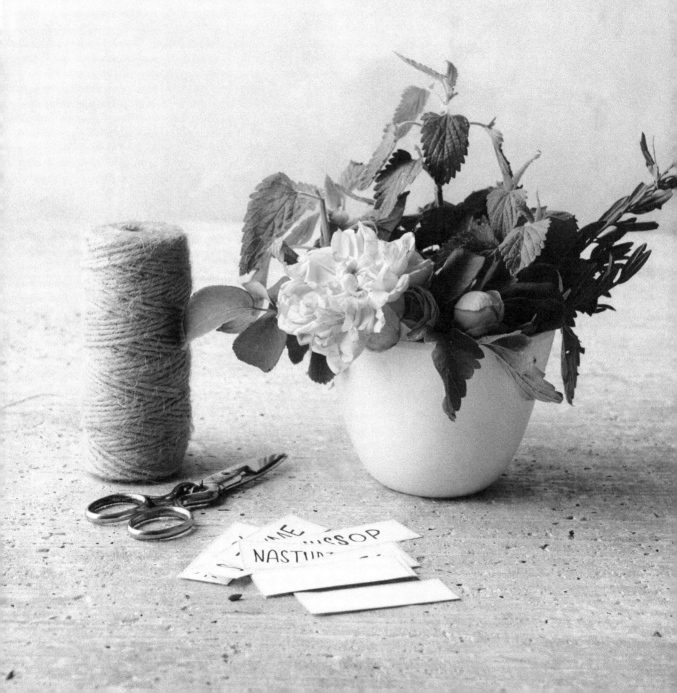

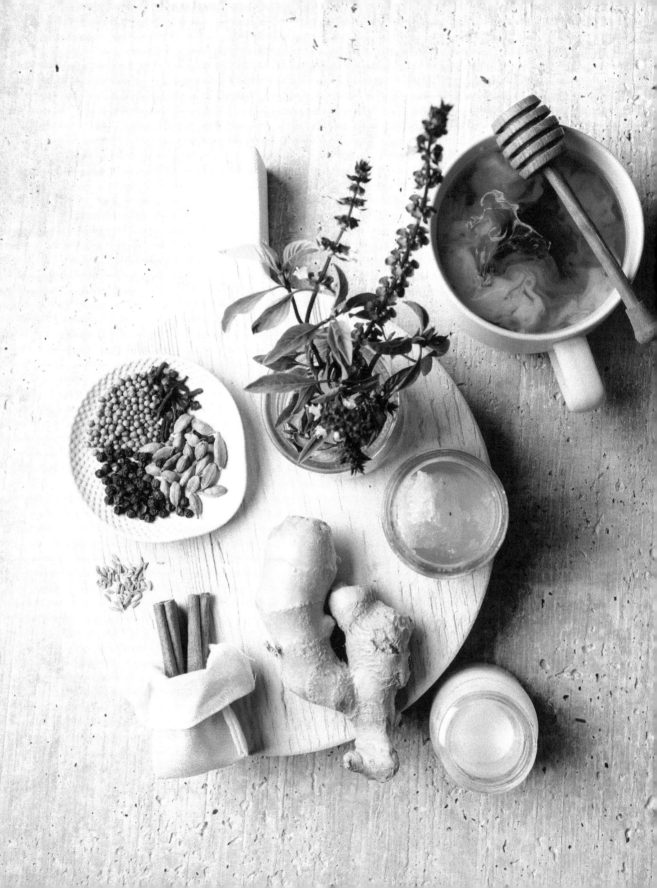

CONTENTS

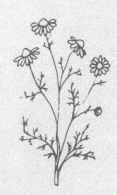

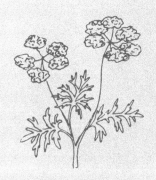

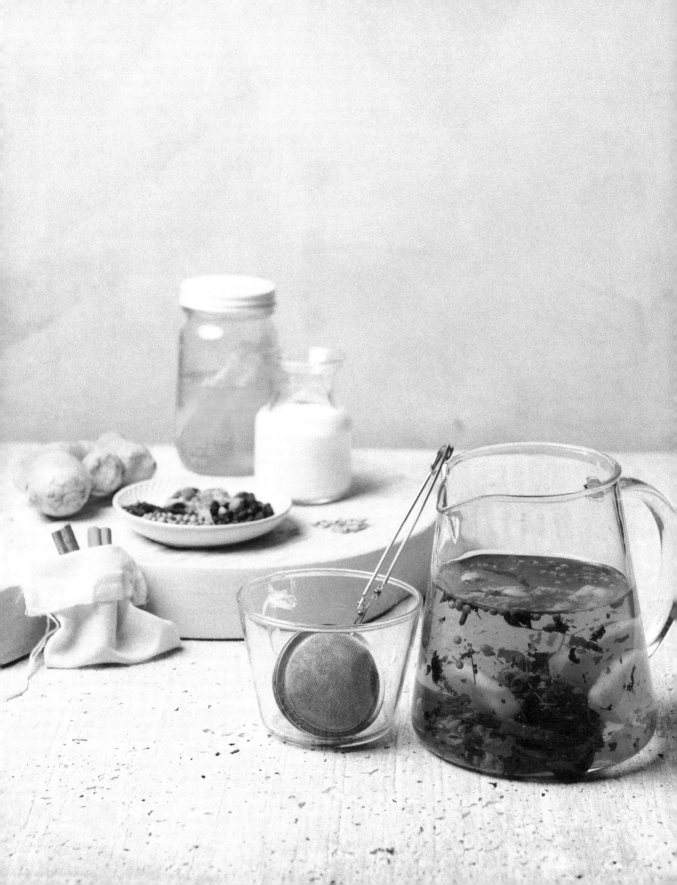

INTRODUCTION

I stumbled into herbs in the early '90s with my sister Maryanne Schwartz when we opened an herb shop at a renaissance festival. At the time, herb people were just figuring out how to offer medicinal herbs for sale, and our learning curve was steep. This led to several years of studying, living, and breathing herbs. A couple years later, we opened another shop called The Herb Basket, where we offered classes every Friday night to our small community. In these classes, we shared the wonderful healing aspects of herbs through soap making, incense making, kitchen cosmetics, herbs for stress, and natural remedies for winter immunity. To keep customers up to date on the classes and goings-on at the shop, we published a bimonthly newsletter. When we eventually sold the shop, that newsletter morphed into *The Essential Herbal*, the magazine that I still publish to this day.

When my sister and I realized the shops were burning us out and made the difficult decision to close them, I couldn't imagine not working with herbs. By then, I was used to being surrounded by jars of herbs, tinctures, potpourris, essential oils, resins, and the fresh plants. Once you've walked outside and gathered yard weeds and a pinch of thyme for an omelet, cooking is never the same. After your child has asked for your own blend of herbal tea that makes her feel better, you know what a superhero feels like. Spreading the word about these very simple things and demystifying herbs and their benefits became my life's work. It's why I publish the magazine, and why I am writing this book—to share the wonderful world of herbs with you, too.

A lot has changed since I first got into herbs. It's hard to believe, looking back, but herbs were considered very much like snake oil. Even culinary herbs were kind of edgy. There were a few good sources of bulk herbs, but for the most part, it was difficult to find them fresh. Most people didn't realize that the dandelions and chickweed in their yards were the same herbs they were reading about in the very few books on herbs that were available. Regulations were nearly impossible to find, making it difficult to follow the rules, so most shops erred on the side of caution. Sellers could not tell a customer what might help a certain ailment.

Interest in herbal medicine has exploded in the past 15 to 20 years, which has fortunately forced every aspect of herbalism to improve. Now you can find fresh herbs at the farmers' market and even your local grocery store, excellent herbal remedies are widely available to purchase, and there are plentiful resources to help you learn how to grow your own herbs. Most people today cook with herbs and may not even realize the healing benefits of doing so!

There are as many herbs as there are plant varieties. It can be completely overwhelming, but that's where this book comes in. My intention is to strip away some of the mystery and show you how you're already using herbs in your daily life. I believe herbal medicine is like home cooking: Just as everyone should be able to prepare a few nutritious meals, everyone should be able to make a few natural remedies for first aid and self-limiting illnesses. You don't need to become a chef or a clinical herbalist to feed and nurture yourself and your family. Having basic knowledge of the healing benefits of herbs is empowering.

In the following pages, I explain the benefits of medicinal herbs, where to look for them, and how to make all kinds of herbal preparations such as teas, tinctures, syrups, oils, salves, pills, baths, and more. You'll learn how to use specific herbs and how to select the best herbs for your needs and constitution. I also include a guide to 30 essential medicinal herbs. I intentionally chose herbs that are easy to find, and a few that are meant to be surprising, such as oats and peppers, in that they are typically considered food instead of medicine. My hope is that by the end of this book, you'll understand that herbs are powerful, all around us, and always our allies in good health.

Let's get started!

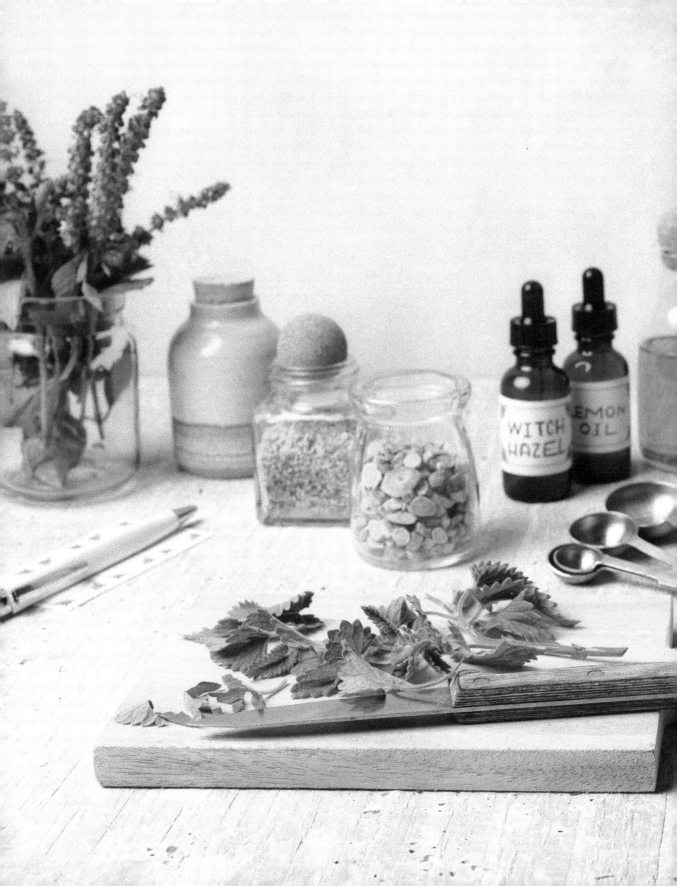

PART I

How Do Herbs Heal?

Plants do so much for us. They provide food, shelter, clothing, and fuel for warmth. They purify the air. In Japan, there is even a practice called *shin-rin-yoku*, or forest bathing, that's based on the idea that just being with plants is healing and restorative.

Plus, plants are medicine.

That old wives' tale "an apple a day keeps the doctor away" is rooted in truth. I consider all plants to be herbs, meaning that they hold immense power to heal our bodies and minds. Herbs contain varying amounts of important vitamins and minerals. They have myriad components that our bodies require to operate smoothly. When you read through the section on Herbs, take note of their incredible properties; many are antibiotic, antifungal, antibacterial, antiviral, and so on. In this section, we get into the nitty-gritty of how herbs heal us in mind and body.

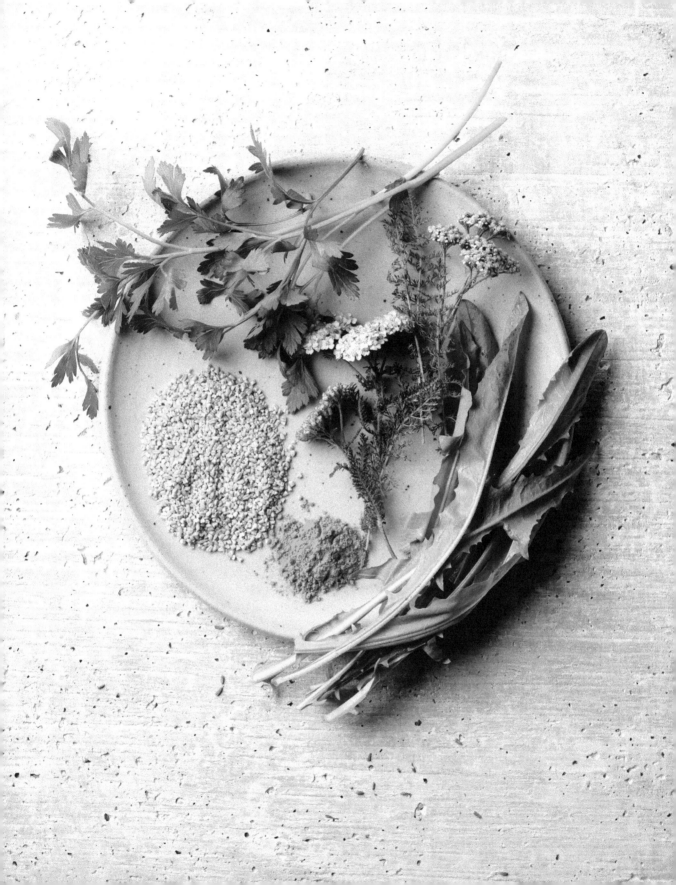

1

What Are Healing Herbs?

Herbs have the amazing capacity to return us to health or help us maintain a healthy state. Quite often, herbs can be the keys that open the door to a healthier, happier life.

Herbs have the power to prevent illness and to provide comfort during illness, injury, and trauma. They can relieve pain, calm the mind, and detoxify the body. Herbs can gently, and without major side effects, work some miracles. They can ease or promote labor and childbirth, help relieve symptoms of lung ailments, improve energy levels, increase circulation, and possibly improve memory and mental sharpness. Some doctors now recommend herbs for lowering blood pressure and cholesterol. With some knowledge and persistence, herbs can take the place of medications of many kinds, including those for acid reflux or insomnia. Best of all, they can help us avoid unnecessary, expensive medical appointments and treatments.

Healing Herbs

So you're probably wondering by now: What *are* the healing herbs and what can they do? The truth is that many of them are probably already stashed in your kitchen somewhere. Take chamomile or mint tea—both are healing herbs! Knowing just three or four herbs and their properties as well as you know that ginger ale helps an upset tummy will make a huge difference in your daily life. There are hundreds of herbal remedies, but here's a taste of a few you might have in (or outside of) your home.

Take oatmeal. It's bulky and keeps us regular, but did you know that it also nourishes the nervous system, helping ease anxiety and stress? Hot peppers, turmeric, and sour cherries are all helpers for the pain of arthritis. Parsley combats bad breath, and those bright green leaves also boost the immune system, stabilize blood sugar, and reduce inflammation. And that oregano on your pizza? It's packed with antioxidants, which help prevent a number of issues related to aging and may even help fight cancer.

It's also important to learn about the weeds outside (and stop killing them with spray!) because they can provide suprising benefits. Wild mint (brightens mood), dandelion (protects the liver), yarrow (antiviral, relaxing), St. John's wort (soothes nerves), mimosa (alleviates grief), and goldenrod (fights allergies) are just a few examples of these wonderful healers. Just outside your door, there are likely to be herbs to heal rashes, insect bites, anxiety, excess bleeding, colds and flu, fevers, sore throats, digestive disorders, and so much more. I'll help you navigate these weeds so you can understand their benefits, and give you ideas for other healing plants to cultivate depending on your needs. Let the medicine making begin!

Benefits of Herbal Medicine

Herbs have been a staple of healing in our house for nearly 30 years. When someone has an ailment, I reach for the herbs first— before going to the drugstore, before calling the doctor.

For example, one summer a family member ran over ground bee nests a few different times on his mower (talk about bad luck!). The first two times, he refused to use any use herbs and was in pain for days. The third time, he finally let me apply mashed plantain (as a poultice; see page 24) to draw out the venom. His pain stopped immediately, and there was no swelling.

During another period in my life, I was caring for a sick sibling who was waiting for an organ transplant. I was warned not to bring any sort of virus or infection into the house because, frankly, it could kill him. For nearly three years, I regularly took elderberry and holy basil to stay healthy, and they worked. Foods and spices eaten mindfully at the right time can make a huge difference.

The best part? Neither of these treatments cost more than a few dollars. The plantain was growing everywhere—I just had to pick it and mix it with water in the food processor. I grow elderberry and holy basil in my yard and had made them into tinctures (see page 20), so vodka was my only expense.

Herbs are safe and gentle (especially those we use as foods and spices), but remember that they are real medicine and should be treated as such. If you take pharmaceutical medications, talk to your doctor and do your research before using herbs. For instance, lemon balm can negatively affect medications used for thyroid issues. Many herbs also thin the blood, which can cause problems if you're taking a blood thinner. If you develop a rash, swelling, or any new symptom while taking the herb, stop using it immediately.

Aside from being inexpensive, herbal remedies can save you time and money over the long run. Remember, many of our ancestors lived their entire lives without setting foot in a doctor's office or hospital! Instead, they ate real food and knew about herbs. With a little forethought and some solid knowledge, herbs make it easy to remain healthy. Simply incorporating them into meals and beverages is a huge step in the right direction. Many herbs have similar functions, so if one isn't convenient or tastes bad, simply exchange it for another.

Most people start by learning how to use herbs to manage symptoms of illnesses that will go away on their own, such as the common cold or respiratory issues. We call those self-limiting illnesses, and they make up a large percentage of (pointless) doctor's visits. We can also learn how to prevent or relieve chronic disease, sometimes even reducing damage already done.

How Are Medicinal Herbs Used?

Although medicinal herbs might seem to be the newest thing, in fact they are the oldest thing! As long as time has been recorded, humans have used plants for healing and nutrition.

There is plenty of evidence of herbal healing in the Bible (although the specific plants are often difficult to ascertain). During the Middle Ages, along with blood-letting and leeches, herbs were the only treatments available. In the Civil War, yarrow was a valued styptic (used to stop bleeding), echinacea helped against infections, pennyroyal was used as an insect repellent, and slippery elm soothed sore throats. As recently as World War II, thyme, foxglove, and peat moss, as well as many other herbs, were purchased from wild crafters who made their living searching woods and meadows for important medicinal plants. There are still people today who harvest wild herbs for a living.

CONVENTIONAL VS. HERBAL MEDICINE

Herbal medicine is different from what many of us are accustomed to with traditional medicine. For instance, when used for chronic or entrenched problems like high blood pressure, GERD, migraines, or reproductive issues, herbal remedies require time and consistency before you'll notice the effects.

However, for minor issues like colds, cramps, or rashes and skin problems, herbs can be as quickly effective as anything you'll find on the drugstore shelf.

A little-known fact is that lots of drugs are actually derived from herbs. One of the best known is the heart medication digitalis, or digoxin, which comes from the foxglove plant. The cancer drug Taxol comes from Pacific yew trees. Of course, there's codeine from poppies, and aspirin from the willow. There's a big difference, though: Pharmaceutical drugs are made by isolating one or two components or chemical constituents from a plant, and then using only those. Pharmaceuticals concentrate that one part of the plant that does that one thing. But plants are so much more than one thing! By contrast, herbal medicine uses all of the components and constituents in the plant, believing that each has a purpose.

It is now quite possible to find a doctor who is learning about herbs and willing to combine them with other medical treatment. I think that's the best of all possible worlds. I'm not suggesting dismissing traditional medicine altogether; rather, I'm encouraging you to understand your options. It is important to get good diagnoses and also to see a doctor if a symptom sticks around too long. Don't avoid getting checked out, and always tell your doctor about any herbs you're taking regularly.

While other parts of the world found ways to incorporate drugs like penicillin and then the sulfa drugs into their natural healing modalities, Americans dropped herbs like hot potatoes and embraced "better living through chemistry." But—surprise, surprise—this wasn't always for the better. Some people got sicker and even died from their medication, despite of years of testing.

In recent decades, people have begun to flock back to herbs in search of the healing knowledge our ancestors took for granted. I remember my own grandfather knew plants only by the nicknames that people from his area used. Even when he didn't know the name, he could go out into the woods or meadows and find a plant that would cure what ailed you. He had a knack for being able to look at a place and say, "I think the plant will be back in there." I am fortunate to have inherited some of his instincts, which makes it easy to find what I need.

Herbs have thousands of components, more than we will ever identify, and they work together to buffer side effects, potentiate other aspects, and, quite honestly, heal in ways we don't yet understand. Using the whole herbs in preparations, as we'll be learning in the next section, makes them safer and more effective at the same time. All those herbs in your kitchen just waiting to help you out will soon become teas, tinctures, elixirs, salves, oils, compresses, and more.

In comparison to pharmaceutical drugs, herbs are extremely safe. The very rare cases of herb-related death are something the entire herb community holds as history. I can think of only three off the top of my head, and one of them was caused by a misidentified herb that was extremely poisonous. The other two were caused by overuse.

There are very few poisonous herbs out there. Herbs labeled as toxic might produce anything from an upset stomach to liver and kidney failure. In more tropical areas, there are more toxic plants. Here are a few things you can do to stay safe:

➤ Always learn foraging from an expert.

➤ Research herbs before using them.

➤ Start at the lowest dose and work up if needed.

Where to Get Them

How you obtain your herbs really depends on where you live—the city, the country, or the suburbs—and your lifestyle. But the three ways to collect herbs are to forage, grow your own, or purchase them.

I live in the country and 80 percent of the herbs I use are wild—also known as weeds! Herbs are plentiful, but being in farm country means that there are many conventional farms around me that use chemicals. I pay attention to their location and when they are spraying, and stay well away from them.

Do not forage herbs that you suspect have been sprayed. In a rural area, hiking trails, unless they are plant conservancies, are safe places to forage and excellent places to learn plant identification.

If you find a safe place to forage, it's important not to gather or taste any herb that you haven't positively identified. Get a couple field guides and study them. Take the field guides and a baggie or basket out into the wild. When an interesting specimen appears, try to determine what the plant is. Take a sprig of it (if there's plenty there) home so you can study it more thoroughly. Once you get a probable ID, put the name of the plant into your browser and do an image search. This will usually tell you if the plant is or isn't what you thought. You don't want to play any guessing games when it comes to foraged plants!

Growing herbs is probably my top choice, and you can do this whether you live on a farm or in a tiny city apartment. You can purchase seeds or starter plants online or at your local nursery. Either way, growing is immensely rewarding.

Another option is purchasing herbs. It's important to use organic herbs in order to avoid chemicals that can be extremely harmful. As consumers, we can use our purchasing power to put an end to the use of these substances that are creating new and ever more resistant pests and plant diseases, not to mention hurting insects, birds, and animals. Fortunately, there are many organic, sustainable, and environmentally conscious people and companies selling beautiful, high-quality herbs. Good-quality herbs have life in them. They don't look like hay. They still have color, scent, and body.

Barks and roots last a couple of years. Aerial herbs—the part of the herbs that grow aboveground but aren't bark, seeds, or fruit—don't last forever. You can extend their usefulness with proper care, such as keeping them in light-blocking containers and storing them in a cool, dry place. When the herbs no longer look, smell, or feel fresh, it's time for the compost pile. After drying, they are considered fresh for about a year if stored well.

Fresh vs. Dried

Fresh herbs picked at the peak of freshness are always preferable. But if these aren't available depending on your location or season, dried is also fine, as long as the quality is there. Another benefit to dried herbs is that they're usually easier to work with. They are easy to store, there's no need to water them, and they take up much less room.

The rule of thumb is that dried is three times stronger than fresh, since the herb becomes concentrated through drying. In volume measurements, one part dry is about equal to three parts fresh herb.

GROW A LITTLE HERB GARDEN

If you have a sunny window, a balcony, or a yard, you can grow herbs. There is nothing like picking your own basil for pesto, snipping a bit of mint for a cup of tea, or even digging up your own horseradish!

If a container garden is necessary due to space restrictions, opt for annual herbs (those that live for only one growing season) and choose the largest container that fits the space. A larger container will allow several plants and also help the herbs retain moisture longer so they survive even if you miss a day of watering.

Now comes the fun part. Decide if the herbs will be culinary, medicinal, or both. Sneak a tomato plant in there, and maybe a pepper or two.

Good culinary choices for beginners are parsley, sage, rosemary, and thyme. Dill is a favorite here, too.

Medicinal herb choices for beginners include holy basil, lemon balm, calendula, mint, and chamomile.

All of these plants can be purchased from your local nurseries, which usually have the best varieties for your region. Grow them as annuals, meaning that they will survive just for one summer and not return next year. If they do come back, it's a bonus.

Although some of these can be grown indoors, herbs are basically weeds and need lots and lots of sun and space. I have poor luck with herbs indoors.

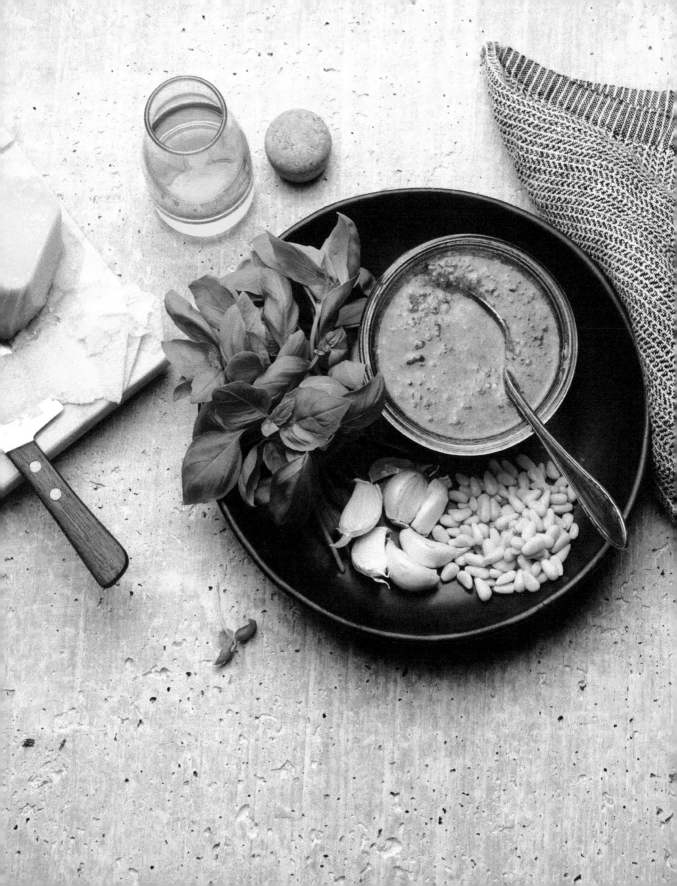

2

How to Use Medicinal Herbs

Herbs have a way of winding their tendrils into everyday life. In fact, you probably ingest more healing herbs than you even realize! But if you want to intentionally incorporate herbs into your routine, there are many simple ways to do so, including:

⚜ Using herbs in cooking and including them as seasoning in all of your meals

⚜ Drinking herbal teas

⚜ Soaking in an herbal bath

⚜ Making and using herbal oils and balms for soft, healthy skin

⚜ Mixing and using tinctures and syrups for well-being

In this chapter, you'll learn formulations and concoctions to mindfully bring herbs into your life.

What You'll Need

Now it's time for the fun part! This chapter covers nine herbal preparations, and you'll need a few supplies at the ready. Don't worry, you don't need anything fancy—my guess is that you have most of these in your kitchen already. Anything else you can easily grab at a craft or kitchen supply store (or even the dollar store!). I also offer DIY alternatives wherever possible.

First things first: Start saving every jar you use! Grab them back out of the recycling bin, wash them, and save them. The same goes for any smallish plastic container that seals, as well as clean zip-top bags. Also, don't throw away old T-shirts. Wash them and cut them into 6-by-6-inch squares to use as filters.

Supplies:

➤ Cutting board

➤ Double boiler

➤ Dropper bottles

➤ Filters (DIY: clean old T-shirts cut into 6-by-6-inch squares)

➤ Funnels in various sizes (DIY: Cut off the top half of a used plastic bottle. These make great funnels and can be used over and over.)

➤ Jars in varying sizes

➤ Knife (a good sharp one)

➤ Labels (big enough to write on)

➤ Measuring cups

➤ Measuring spoons

➤ Muslin bags for compresses (DIY: material from clean, old cotton or flannel sheets)

➤ Scale. If you find that you really enjoy making salves and balms and want to make any quantity, the ingredients should be weighed. A decent scale is always a good investment.

➤ Strainers, both fine and regular mesh

➤ Tea infusers (or tea balls), one small (for individual cups) and one large (for pots of tea). The perforated metal balls are most common, but you can also find these made of silicone in different, fun shapes, as well as other types of infusers.

Non-herbal ingredients:

➤ Alcohol, typically vodka (190-proof is excellent, 151-proof is the next choice, and 100-proof also works)

➤ Beeswax (sold in craft stores and health food stores)

➤ Olive oil

These are the basic supplies you need to get started. When we get to the individual sections, I suggest additional options, but you can generally make do without those. After a little practice, you can also come up with your own way of doing things—that's part of the fun.

For many years, these were the only tools I used. As time went by, I acquired a distiller to make hydrosols and essential oils, a press specifically made to extract all of the oil or liquid from an infusion, and a couple magic choppers. I love them, but I managed for a long time without them.

Two other things you'll need are time and space. Keep in mind that these are healing preparations and therefore you want to pay attention to your intentions and your mood while creating them. Try to pour some love and care into these concoctions as you work. Clear a space. Put on some good music. Take your time and enjoy the process. Certainly, this isn't always possible. Sometimes the kid is in the bedroom hacking away, and you're tired, and there's a bit of vomit streaked down your back. Of course, you'll do what you need to do depending on the situation.

But if you can carve out some dedicated time to prepare an herbal medicine arsenal that's ready and waiting for the next cold, flu, or upset stomach, it's worth it. The first time someone asks for your special tea or you can produce a healing tincture with the snap of a finger, it's a great feeling.

Herbal Teas

Herbal teas are one of the easiest and most pleasant ways to incorporate herbs into your daily life. Sometimes they are called tisanes; when only a single herb is used for a tea, it is called a simple tea. But most people just call them herbal teas.

Herbal teas are differentiated from the teas made from the plant *Camellia sinensis*, which include black, green, oolong, and white teas. These all come from a single plant, which is technically an herb that contains caffeine! What we consider to be herbal teas do not have caffeine, so that's the main distinction.

Lots of people are only vaguely aware of the medicinal properties of the teas that they've come to regularly enjoy. Herbal teas are one of the gentlest means of taking medicinal herbs. Many of them can be given to children—my daughter still remembers the chamomile tea parties we'd have during scary thunderstorms or other stressful times. Twenty-plus years later, chamomile is still a favorite tisane that's always in her cupboard.

Teas were my gateway herbs. After spending a winter reading various herb books, I spent the spring, summer, and fall gathering sprigs and petals of every possible herb I could use for tea, pinching bits from gardens of friends or leaping from the car to run across a meadow for something. I dried them on a screen and mixed them together in a big jar. I added some purchased stevia leaves, cinnamon chips, and licorice root, and shook it up. We brewed the concoction by the cup. Each cup was different, and there wasn't a bad one in the bunch.

There are a couple of different brewing methods. When using the more tender parts of the plant, like the leaves, the herbs are infused. This involves pouring hot water

DRYING YOUR HERBS

Drying herbs is simple, and there are lots of ways to do it. The main thing is to keep them away from moisture and direct sunlight. I like to lay clean bedsheets on my attic floor and spread out the herbs so they aren't touching each other. There's dry heat and no air-conditioning, and I keep the curtains closed. After a few days, the herbs are dried perfectly.

Things like berries, roots, or bark take a long time to dry and need circulation, so having a few old window screens around is perfect. Place the botanicals on the screen and elevate it so that air can get underneath.

You can also put small quantities of herbs in bunches, with rubber bands around the stems to hold them together, and hang them until dry. Be sure there aren't too many stems, though, or the center can mold. Hang the herb bunches away from direct light.

If humidity is a problem in your house, try spreading the herbs in a shallow layer on a cookie sheet and placing in a warm oven set on the lowest setting. If it's a gas oven, just the pilot light will work. Depending on the herbs and how much is on the pan, they will be fine in there overnight. Stir them up in the morning to see if they're dry. If they're almost dry, allow them to finish at room temperature. If they're still pretty damp, return them to the oven. When done, immediately seal them in a jar or baggie so they don't absorb moisture.

The goal with dried herbs is to keep the leaves as intact as possible in order to preserve the essential oils and other components. You can remove the leaves from the stems prior to drying. If I'm in a hurry, I will strip the leaves from the stems after drying (a little trickier), or even just leave them on the stems until it's time to use them. Dried herbs are easier to store without the stems.

Store dried herbs away from light in a cool, dark location.

over the herbs (which you can place in a tea ball or tea bag) and letting it steep for 5 to 15 minutes before straining.

Don't confuse this technique with the recent popularity of the word *infusion*, as in "herbal infusions." This refers to a very concentrated beverage made using one ounce of dried herb in a quart of water and steeping it overnight. There are only a handful of plants suited to this method, including vitamin- and mineral-laden herbs like stinging nettle, red clover, and oats.

As a general guideline, use a teaspoon of dried herb or herb blend or a tablespoon of fresh herbs per one cup (8 ounces) of tea. That said, the measurement isn't critical with tea. I usually go over because I keep adding things!

Teas made with denser bark, seeds, or roots are decocted. I'll often make up a decoction of wild cherry bark, licorice root, fennel seeds, and perhaps a couple of other roots, depending on the purpose. To decoct, simmer the herb in water for an extended period of time, which can be from 15 minutes to several hours depending on the herb. The harder the material, the more heat and time needed to extract the properties and flavors.

In terms of which herbs to use for your teas, a lot depends on where you live and what is available. Some good herbs to try are mint, chamomile, sage, thyme, hibiscus, jasmine, passionflower, or lemon balm. Sprinkle in some rose petals. Raspberry and blueberry leaves add flavor and have useful components.

For a simple, relaxing tea, try blending chamomile, passionflower, and lemon balm.

To soothe a cold and sore throat, try sage, thyme, and elderberry with a licorice root stir stick.

Upset tummy? Ginger tea with a little spearmint can work wonders.

Teas are especially valuable for comfort and calming.

Syrups

Making syrups is a simple way to preserve herbs using inexpensive ingredients. Some syrups are tasty enough to drizzle over ice cream, crepes, or into cocktails or shrubs. Syrups can take the most horrendous flavor and make it palatable enough for a child to enjoy. Horehound is a good example: It's an acquired taste, at best (although there are people who like it), but it's terrific for soothing coughs and a variety of upper-respiratory issues. Mixing it with some sugar, honey, or molasses helps the medicine go right down.

To make syrup, you'll need a pan, strainer, measuring cups, funnel, bottles, and a spoon.

Start with a strong herbal tea that has been simmered down to reduce by about half. Next, add either 2 parts sugar (1 cup tea, 2 cups sugar) or an equal amount of honey or molasses (1 cup tea, 1 cup honey or molasses). I generally use sugar because it's inexpensive and I always have it in the house. Stir to be sure the sugar (or honey or molasses) is dissolved, bring to a rolling boil, and continue to boil for about three minutes. Cool, bottle, and cap.

Syrups can keep for up to a year in the refrigerator. If you want to store without refrigeration, concentrate the infusion more by simmering it down to about one-third the original quantity, and add ¼ cup 100-proof vodka for every 1 cup of syrup (resulting in 12.5 percent alcohol content).

This alcohol content is not much when taken by the teaspoon, but be aware of it for children and pregnant women.

Elderberry syrup is a must every year for winter health, and I share a recipe in the elder section (see page 95).

A staple syrup in our household is one that's great for soothing mucus in the throat and chest. The main ingredients are osha, elecampane, ginger, licorice root, some mullein, California poppy, and horehound. I simmer the roots separately until the liquid is almost reduced by half, then add the more delicate herbs for the rest of the simmer. I then continue as described above, adding whatever sweetener I prefer and alcohol if desired.

A simple ginger syrup is good to have around because once it's in the cabinet, you'll be reaching for it to add to teas, baked goods, stir-fries, and so much more. Blackstrap molasses makes a tasty and nourishing base.

In the spring, violet, rose, and dandelion syrups are fun and beautiful to make. Those work best with a sugar base and some lemon, which allow the gorgeous colors to come through.

Oils

Infused herbal oils are made by soaking herbs in a vegetable or nut oil for an extended period, with or without heat. It is important to mention that this is completely different from an essential oil.

Many different oils can be infused. Olive is the most common because it's easy to find, affordable, and great for the skin. Sweet almond oil is often found as an ingredient in older herbals, but it tends to go rancid quickly if not refrigerated. Apricot, avocado, sesame, hazelnut, sunflower, and jojoba (technically a wax, making it extremely shelf stable) are also good options.

Most herbal oil infusions are used topically in salves, balms, lotions, soaps, and massage oils. They can be used as culinary oils, but that requires extreme caution, as any moisture at all can result in botulism.

There are several methods for making herbal oils. The key is to make sure that no water is introduced into the oil. The moisture that is in the plant material must be allowed to evaporate freely or the oil will develop mold. Additionally, all plant material must be completely covered by oil to avoid mold.

COOKING WITH HERBS FOR HEALTH

"Let food be thy medicine and medicine be thy food."
—HIPPOCRATES

Herbs pack a lot of value. A sprinkling of thyme, a tablespoon of basil pesto, a teaspoon of parsley, or some sesame seeds on a bagel—all add incredible flavor and are powerhouses of nutrients and protective properties.

Cooking with herbs doesn't need to be involved. One of the first classes we gave at our shop was an herb tasting. We had crackers, butter, cream cheese, and about 10 culinary herbs: chives, tarragon, basil, rosemary, sage, parsley, chervil, thyme, cilantro, and paprika. The attendees simply put a dab of butter or cheese on a cracker and added a sprig of an herb, learning about each herb as they snacked. They left feeling more confident about using culinary herbs at home.

To begin cooking with herbs, start small, meaning one serving at a time. That way, if it isn't great, you haven't ruined a big meal. A scrambled egg is the perfect place to add a little thyme, parsley, and a splash of salsa with cilantro. That's how I learned, and now I can't imagine cooking a dish without something green or spicy to jazz it up and bring out the flavor.

DOSAGE

The vast majority of herbs, when used with a little knowledge, are gentle and don't require dosages as precise as medicinal drugs. The dosage generally depends on the herb, the individual, the energetics (covered in the next chapter), and the issue or ailment being addressed.

When using a new herb, the best thing to do is start with a small amount. If it's a tea, start with a cup and see how you feel. With a tincture, 12 to 15 drops is a good start. For syrup, a teaspoon or two will do. On the rare occasions when I get sick, these rules go out the window because I know how different herbs affect me after years of trial and error. You may find me wandering around with a box of tissues, swigging from a bottle of elderberry syrup, and simultaneously pouring it into my giant mug of ginger, honey, and lemon tea. Over time, I've gained a deep understanding of what works for me.

Taking too much of an herb *can* result in minor diarrhea (similar to eating too much broccoli or cabbage), sleeplessness or sleepiness, or something similarly benign. If you don't experience these symptoms, feel free to slowly increase your dose if desired.

To determine a child's dosage, consider their weight. We generally assume an average adult weight to be about 150 pounds. If the adult dose is 30 drops, then a 30-pound child would get one-fifth of the adult dose, or six drops. Another helpful trick is using one drop per year of age up to age 12. As mentioned above, herbs are not as exacting as pharmaceutical drugs, but it's always smart to err on the side of caution when it comes to children.

Specific dosage guidelines are difficult to find. You can consult with an herbalist if you're feeling unsure and looking for more guidance. And always speak with an herbalist or doctor when working with a chronic condition or illness.

To make infused oil, you'll need a large glass measuring cup, a strainer, a jar for storing, and, if using fresh herbs, cheesecloth.

The easiest method is to start with dried herbs in oil using gentle heat. The oven on the lowest setting or a slow cooker equipped with a low setting work very well, and a jar of oil and herbs sitting in a south-facing window is great. I'm always in a hurry, so it's the slow cooker overnight for me. The oven would also be overnight, and the window could take a few weeks.

If you want to use fresh herbs, which can be tricky, they should be well wilted to lessen the water content. After mixing the herbs into the oil, cover the jar with several layers of cheesecloth to allow evaporation until the infusion is finished. The infusion is done when it has taken on the scent and/or color of the herb, usually after at least two weeks.

Many years ago I made a gallon of jewelweed oil and didn't wilt it or allow it to evaporate, keeping the bottle sealed. It looked great, but when I opened the jug in the spring, it was putrid.

When the oil is finished, strain out the herbs. I have a favorite method for straining: using 6-inch squares of material from old T-shirts. Line a mesh strainer with one of these squares and set it over a large (2-quart) glass measuring cup. Then pour the oil and herbs slowly through it. Squeeze the material to get all the good oil into the cup. Pour the oil into a jar or bottle, cap, and label.

You can also infuse solid oils like shea, coconut, cocoa butter, soy, and mango butter. Liquefy them with gentle heat and then introduce the herbs. On warm, sunny days, you can put them in the heat of the sun until they are liquid and then add your herbs. After several hours, put the oil in the refrigerator and keep it there until you need it. At that time, heat the oil to liquid again, strain the plant material, and use.

In the following sections, you'll see how you can mix oils into a variety of preparations like salves, balms, and massage oils to add a healing herbal component.

Salves

Salves are emollient and healing blends of herbal oils. You can make all-purpose salves for any skin problem, antiseptic salves for healing wounds; drawing salves for pulling out splinters, venom, and infections; salves for chest rubs; or salves for sore muscles. They can even be made as a pleasant hand softener or lip balm. Salves, lip balms, and the more solid lotion bar are all basically the same thing. The only difference is the amount of beeswax used. Once you learn this skill, it comes in handy for all sorts of things—salve variations can be used for hair pomade, diaper rash cream, and even furniture polish!

To add herbs to salves, the herbs are first infused in oil, then blended with beeswax.

Vegan options for wax include bayberry, candelilla, or a high percentage of cocoa butter in place of wax.

Here are some general starting points:

SALVE 1 part wax to 8 parts oil

LIP BALM 1 part wax to 4 parts oil

LOTION BARS 1 part wax to 2 parts oil

To make a salve, you'll need a double boiler (or a microwave and glass measuring cup), a stainless steel spoon, jars, and labels.

Start with about one-fourth of the oil to be used and mix it with the wax. Heat the mixture to melt the wax. You can do this in either a double boiler or the microwave. If using the microwave, heat in 30-second increments, stirring after each. Either way, continue until the wax is completely melted. Be sure the remaining oil is at room temperature, then add it to the wax mixture. This prevents heating all of the oil to the melting point of the wax. But don't worry, you can't really ruin a salve. You simply add more oil or more wax until you have the right consistency.

Tinctures

Tinctures may sound scientific and intimidating, but as it turns out, this folk method couldn't be easier. Tinctures are simply plants infused in alcohol for a period of time until the liquid becomes much like a very concentrated tea. Fresh herbal properties can be well preserved in a tincture with almost no work and just a little time.

Tinctures are simple to make and a perfect way to preserve medicinal herbs.

I always keep chamomile tincture around. My daughter was anxious as a child and had difficulty falling asleep, and I found that chamomile was just the thing. I also keep a blend of holy basil and mimosa flower on hand for emotionally draining situations, when I can't see the forest for the trees.

You'll need a knife or scissors, a cutting board, alcohol (typically vodka), jars, and labels. Wilt the herbs to get rid of excess moisture and then use a good quality-vodka (150-proof is my go-to). Some people prefer whiskey, rum, or brandy; it's just a matter of taste. Fill a jar with chopped herbs. Cover with your alcohol of choice. Leave at room temperature for six weeks, shaking the jar daily (or when you remember). After six weeks, strain the mixture and your tincture is ready for use.

Some people put their herbs in a food processor first. Some people shake their jars every day.

If you don't need to use the tincture right away, it is fine to leave it unstrained for years. In fact, tinctures keep for many years just as they are, strained or with the herbs left in the alcohol.

To use a tincture, start at a low dose and see how it works. Mix it with a swallow of water or juice. Tinctures don't always taste great, so get it over with quickly. Some people choose to put tinctures straight under their tongues, but in my opinion, there's no

LABELING

Always label your preparations! Do this as soon as you're done making them. Skipping this step is how I ended up with my famous shelf of unknown remedies. There are still times when I'll be called away in the middle of preparing something and forget to label what I added, and the memory instantly fades. The second there's even a fleeting doubt, it's too late, and you can't be certain what went into your preparation.

Your labels should include:

NAME OF THE REMEDY

DATE MADE

INGREDIENTS

INSTRUCTIONS FOR USE

Start a notebook from the moment you begin creating formulas. Write down the steps as you work so you know how to re-create things. There's nothing worse than making the world's best-ever tea blend and then forgetting what went into it.

If stored in the refrigerator, most preparations can last about a year. Without preservatives, that's a good rule of thumb.

HARVESTING HERBS

We will examine individual herbs later in the book, but here are a few tips to keep in mind as you begin harvesting. Before starting, do your research to understand which part of the plant is used. It is best to use clippers, but your fingers will work fine, too (but most herbies I know have perpetually stained fingers throughout the summer!). Choose only the healthiest plants.

- Gather at least 100 feet from a roadway, and only where you know pesticides and weed killers have not been used.
- Get permission from the property owner if you are foraging.
- Never forage in a protected area or plant conservancy.
- Choose plants that are at or just before their peak, with leaves and flowers that have no blemishes.
- If possible, wait until the dew has dried.
- Gather fragrant essential oil–producing plants before the hottest point of the day.
- *Never* wipe out a stand of plants. Pick no more than 10 percent of what's there. If it is the lone stand, consider leaving it until next year. If there are seeds on what you're picking, leave the seeds behind.
- Learn the list of endangered and at-risk plants in your area (UnitedPlantSavers.org is a great resource) and be a good steward.
- Process the gathered herbs immediately for the best quality.
- Dry herbs as you go. If you're like me and go out for long stretches of time, you can use large, loosely woven baskets and fill them only halfway. Give the herbs a turn a couple of times a day, and they'll dry in the basket.

need to suffer like that. You can also mix a dose into a cup of tea (even herbal tea) or juice.

Regarding the alcohol in tinctures: The typical dosage is less than a teaspoon of alcohol. Most sources will say that this is equivalent to the naturally occurring alcohol content in a ripe banana. I never hesitated to give a few drops mixed in juice to my toddler. As long as the herb is safe to use during pregnancy, this amount of alcohol shouldn't be a problem. Still, I would never suggest that someone who cannot have alcohol should use tinctures. There are lots of other good ways to ingest herbs, so why risk it?

If alcohol isn't an option for you for whatever reason, you can substitute glycerin using three parts glycerin to one part water. It isn't quite as effective, and the tinctures last only for a year or so, but it is a decent substitute.

Pills

Pills (or pastilles) are another remedy that is very easy and inexpensive to make. There's nothing in the pills except the herb and whatever liquid or moistener is used to form the pill. You can use any herb or combination of herbs, and, with practice, the pills can be made to be quite tasty. I particularly like to use them for sore throats.

To make pills, combine freshly powdered herbs with a liquid to form a thick, firm paste.* The paste is then rolled into balls, which may or may not be flattened into a lozenge shape, and then dried. These come in handy for children—the pills can be made smaller or larger depending on what the child can hold in his or her mouth and how much herb is desired. To take the pill, hold it in your mouth until it breaks apart and can be swallowed.

You'll need a bowl, knife, spoon, jars or tins, and labels. It's very important to finely powder the herbs. I like to use a coffee grinder and then put the powder through a mesh strainer to remove any larger bits. You can also purchase powdered herbs, but be aware that powders lose their vitality very quickly. It's always best to keep herbs as whole as possible until use.

Next, choose your liquid. Honey is usually my first choice, but you can also use tea, glycerin, coconut oil, or a medicinal syrup you've made. Start with two parts herbal powder to one part liquid. Add the liquid a bit at a time, and knead the mixture very well, adding more liquid as needed. Get similarly sized pieces by rolling the "dough" into a log and cutting off short lengths. Dry thoroughly. Dry pills should be shelf stable for several months, but I stick them in the refrigerator or freezer out of habit. They'll basically last forever if frozen.

Another easy way to make a pill is to get empty capsules and fill them with powdered herbs. These are meant to be swallowed and are sometimes the only way to get someone to take a bitter herb!

The mixture before drying is called an electuary, which can be added to or used to make herbal teas.

Baths

Herbs in the tub can do a lot. As a child, I remember my mother putting me in the kitchen sink full of oatmeal water, probably for measles or the chicken pox. It was so soothing. A cup of vinegar steeped with roses poured into a tepid bath is a wonder for sunburn. Comfrey and Epsom salts after too much physical activity relaxes muscles and helps achy joints. The list goes on and on. A nice herbal bath can be so healing.

Baths are made in much the same way as teas that are formulated to drink, but they are combined to soothe or nourish the skin. Sometimes you can drink the same concoction that will be used for bathing, and honey can even be part of the deal.

I often hear instructions to hang a muslin bag filled with herbs from the faucet while drawing the bath. That really doesn't work well, though. I prefer to fill a half gallon pitcher with very hot water, then submerge a muslin bag filled with the herbs in the water while running a bath. It makes a strong "tea" that you can then pour into the bath. No muslin bag? No worries. Place the herbs in the center of a washcloth, bind the corners with a rubber band, and make your "tea" that way.

You can put additions like oatmeal, powdered milk, or salt directly into the bag, or in the water separately. Just don't clog the drain.

Herbs for the bath can be used fresh or dried. Good choices are comfrey root and leaf, calendula flowers, roses, lavender, chamomile, mint, yarrow, plantain, jewelweed, rosemary, thyme, elderflower, chickweed, seaweed, and sage.

Poultices

Poultices are used to treat issues by applying herbs directly onto the skin. They are typically, but not always, used for external issues. They may be used to soothe or calm rashes, and are also valuable for drawing out toxins, stings, and splinters. Making herbal poultices can be as simple as chewing up a leaf and putting the wet, mashed herb onto an insect bite or wound. Or it can be as involved as heating a mixture of herbs in oil and applying it to the skin, covered with layers of material.

Tea bag poultices are easy and quick, and people commonly use them without thinking of them as poultices. For instance, years ago it felt like I might be developing a stye on my eye, so I brewed up two tea bags in one cup, one chamomile and one echinacea, to put on the affected eye. As one tea bag cooled, I would replace it on my eye with the other. Rotating the tea bags stopped the stye or infection from getting a foothold.

"Spit poultices" are hurried preparations made in the field. For instance, for yellow jacket or wasp stings, an instant remedy is a plantain leaf chewed and applied to the sting after removing the stinger. It provides immediate relief, and if done promptly, draws out the venom before damage occurs.

I once had a blocked salivary gland. After spending a good deal of time finding the gland, I made small, half-moon-shaped poultices in heat-sealable tea bags. I filled them with a blend of plantain, chickweed, and kaolin clay, and they successfully pulled the little "stone" out.

A mustard plaster placed on the chest would be considered a poultice, as would the old-time practice of chopping and cooking large amounts of onions and spreading them as hot as could be borne on the chest. Both of these have a layer of cloth between them and the skin to prevent skin irritation. They're both commonly used to increase circulation and loosen chest congestion.

Compresses

Most everyone has used a hot or cold compress after a muscle injury. Herbal compresses are similar but have the added healing properties of herbs. They can be prepared for use at different temperatures, depending on the purpose. Hot compresses are used for muscular pains, cramping, and drawing out infections. Most other issues call for room-temperature or cool compresses.

Making a compress is very easy. Use a nice thick washcloth, or a hand towel for larger areas.

1. Make a very strong herbal tea in a quantity that will allow you to saturate the cloth.

2. Soak tea into the cloth and wring it out.

3. Place the soaked cloth on the affected area for 15 to 30 minutes.

4. Repeat as needed.

If you prefer a cold compress, place the soaked cloth in the freezer briefly (take it out before it freezes). This is faster than waiting for the tea to cool down. Teas brewed for compresses can be refrigerated or frozen and reheated when needed. Be sure to mark any frozen teas like you would other preparations. It's no fun to find containers of herbal ice cubes and have no clue as to what they might contain.

Here are some of my go-to compresses:

SUNBURN Black tea with lavender and rose petals. This should be used as a cool, but not cold, compress.

MUSCLE SPRAINS OR STRAINS WITH NO BROKEN SKIN Arnica with comfrey and Epsom salts, applied warm.

GENERAL RASH Chamomile, applied cool or at room temperature to soothe and calm the skin.

ACHING OR NERVE PAIN Lemon balm with St. John's wort, used either very warm or very cold, perhaps alternating.

ECZEMA Plantain, chickweed, calendula, and lavender applied at room temperature.

PLANT RASHES (POISON IVY, OAK, SUMAC) Yarrow with jewelweed and plantain applied as a cool compress.

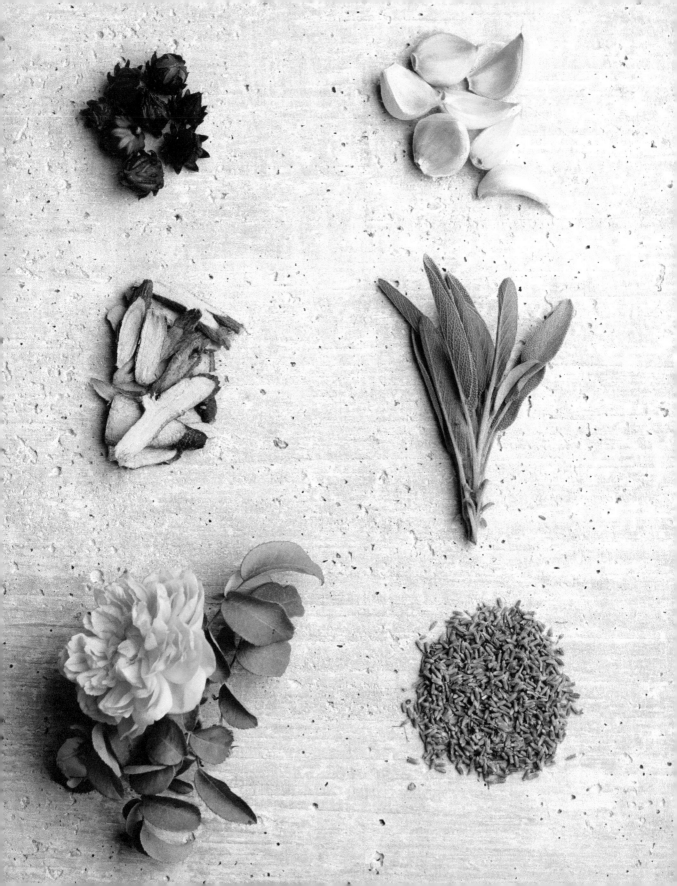

3

Selecting the Best Herbs for You

In this chapter, we discuss the different classifications for humans, herbs, and illnesses. In traditional Western herbalism, this system is called herbal energetics. We are all so very different and unique, but we can be classified into four main constitutions that describe our general physical state. While your constitution can change throughout your life, it's the basis of who you are right now. When treating an illness, it's important to match the herb, illness, and individual energetically. For instance, some herbs are very drying. Let's say a person with a dry constitution is experiencing a tight, dry cough. Giving them a drying herb would only make the situation worse. Instead, we would give them something that will moisten and ease the cough. This is the basic framework of energetics.

Energetics of Individuals

Most cultures have a healing tradition that helps us make the connection between a person's constitution and what kind of herbs will help bring them back to balance. Examples from around the world include Ayurveda, traditional Chinese medicine, the Native American Medicine Wheel, and Southern folk herbalism. These are all essentially different forms of energetics. In this chapter, we'll examine the philosophy of traditional Western medicine energetics, which is over 100 years old and a melding of many traditions.

Individual energetics refers to one's constitution, which is the general condition of the body. It is important to choose the right herb energy for the constitution of the person. Determine your own constitution by pondering the following list. For some people, it will be as clear as a bell, while for others it may require some examination and thought.

My own constitution is damp and neutral temperature (neither hot or cold), tending toward lax.

Some of the things that lead me to this classification are my ability to sweat on cue and the feeling that it might be possible to die from humidity (damp). I have many hot and cold markers, so that lands me in the neutral territory. If nobody forces me to move around and do things, I'll probably take a couple naps and not get dressed for the day (lax).

Here are the types:

Cool/cold:

- Quiet
- Would like another sweater, please
- Pale complexion
- Cold hands and feet
- Sluggish or inactive

Warm/hot:

- Outspoken
- Usually feels warm
- Blushes easily
- Always doing something active, can be hyper
- Healthy appetite

Damp

- Oily skin and hair
- Retains water easily
- Sweats easily and freely
- Does not like humidity
- Prone to congestion or runny nose
- Ankles may swell easily

Dry

- Brittle nails, hair breaks easily

- Dry skin and scalp

- Itchy

- Prone to dry cough and throat

- Creaky joints

- Prone to constipation

Tense

- Nervous or irritable, easily rattled

- Tight, painful muscles

- Headaches

- Too busy

Lax/Relaxed

- Prone to depression (physical and emotional)

- Sleepy, difficult to wake

- Sluggish, stagnant

- At its worst, may mean loss of muscle control

Each of us individually falls somewhere on the scale of the three categories below. We all land somewhere between hot and cold, damp and dry, and tense and lax. Those things all change from time to time, but we *tend* toward one side or the other unless drastic life changes occur. For instance, I have seen a warm, damp person become cool and dry after chemotherapy.

If neither type in one category applies, or if they seem equal, you may have a neutral, or balanced, constitution, and that's a good thing. Balance is the goal in health, as it is in all things. Our constitution is part of who we are through heredity and ethnicity, so we can't change it completely, but we can make changes through herbs, food, and lifestyle that move us toward balance.

Personally, I notice that weight changes, age, activity level, and eating habits alter my constitution. Weight gain can bring lots of water retention and bogginess to my

COOL ~ COLD	NEUTRAL	WARM ~ HOT

DAMP	NEUTRAL	DRY

TENSE	NEUTRAL	LAX

body, causing me to perspire more often and lean toward the damp type. Losing weight and upping activity, along with eating lots of good fresh fruits and vegetables, can return me to a more balanced constitution with more control of moisture, tone, and temperature. Similarly, someone with a cold, dry constitution can sometimes neutralize that with hydration, exercise (to warm the muscles and organs), and consumption of warming, moist foods.

For home herbalists, knowing your baseline constitution is valuable. It helps you understand the foods and herbs that can steer you closer to the center, as well as the foods and herbs that you want to avoid. Understanding our own constitution and that of those close to us enables us to choose the correct herb for the individual.

Energetics of Herbs

Now that you understand the types of constitution/tissue states, you can select herbs that correspond to each one. Yes, herbs have energetics, too! The trick is to work with herbs that promote balance in the body. For instance, a cooling herb would be called for in a hot state, a drying herb for a damp state, or a relaxing herb for too much tension. Here are some common examples:

COOLING watermelon, lettuce, raspberry leaf, hibiscus, lavender

WARMING cayenne, ginger, basil, garlic, cinnamon, black pepper

MOISTURIZING licorice, marshmallow root, plantain, okra, purslane, slippery elm

DRYING sage, osha, turmeric, tea, yarrow, goldenrod

TONING (INVIGORATES TONE AND TIGHTNESS) yarrow, witch hazel, tea, rose, blackberry leaf, lady's mantle

RELAXING valerian, lemon balm, hops, catnip, chamomile, lavender

Within the various types, many herbs have different actions. For instance, when it comes to relaxing herbs, chamomile very gently calms anxiety, milky oat seed supports the nervous system, passionflower helps with circular thinking that creates tension, and skullcap relieves stress and mental exhaustion. Herbs work in different and powerful ways.

Furthermore, the taste of herbs and foods also corresponds to the energetics of herbs. The taste of an herb reinforces its action. Here are the tastes most often used in herbal healing, with some examples:

SWEET (WARM, DAMP) cardamom, nutmeg, anise, sesame seeds

SALTY (COLD, DRY) seaweed, vinegar, celery, soy sauce, nettles

PUNGENT (HOT, DRY) horseradish, mustard, paprika, cumin

SPICY (WARM, DRY) cinnamon, cloves, ginger, holy basil

SOUR (COOL, DRY) lemon, sumac, tamarind, fermented foods

ASTRINGENT (DRY) tea, oregano, parsley, cranberries

BITTER (COLD, DAMP) hops, mugwort, citrus peel, dandelion, gentian, yellow dock

In choosing herbs, keep in mind that the goal is always to move from an excess of a particular constitutional element toward balance. If an illness exhibits cold and wet symptoms, you want to respond with herbs that are warm/hot and dry to balance them out.

Let's say someone is hot, dry, and tense in constitution, and this is causing issues with constipation. You'd want to choose cooling, demulcent, or moistening herbs that tend to have a sweet taste. Licorice root, slippery elm, and marshmallow root would all be helpful for this person.

If we combine the herbs that will work in balance with the person's constitution and the tastes that affect that action, we can be better assured that we're choosing the correct herb for the situation.

Energetics of Illnesses

Many years ago my sister and I were on a road trip and chatting about how difficult it is to accurately describe pain to the doctor. At some point she said hers was a round, sweet pain. We laughed for about 10 miles after that one.

Looking back, I see that we were onto something, we just weren't using the terminology of a recognized tradition. The truth is that illnesses have energetics, too.

Once you become familiar with the energetics of humans and herbs, it becomes clear how they correlate to the symptoms of an illness and how best to approach and treat that illness. One way to look at it is that the illness presents itself by demonstrating in what way the body is out of balance. Heat needs to be cooled; damp requires drying. Simple yet true.

Consider the language we use to describe an illness or its symptoms. How often do we use the terms that describe the tissue states, or variations of the terms? "This cold is stuck in my chest," or "My back is so tense that it's got my head aching, too." It's already how we think about illness. Now we just need to put it all together.

Let's say your child has a weeping skin rash (damp). Your goal will be to dry it up so it can heal. You wouldn't put oil or any kind of barrier over it, because it needs contact with the air to dry. If you had dry, painful patches such as brush burns or cracked hands, you wouldn't reach for a drying treatment like a drawing clay poultice. You would likely know all this instinctively, without having to think about the energetics involved.

Eventually, this system of healing becomes second nature. I encourage people to think about how much they use this system without realizing it, then go from

STORAGE

When it comes to storing herbal preparations, first and foremost date your jars! Since they are not chemically preserved, you want to throw them out after a year (unless they are obviously past their prime before then). Tinctures are an exception and can last for up to 10 years if properly stored. But a year is a good guideline for most everything else. Here are some storage tips:

* Use bottles or jars that have a dark color, such as amber or blue. This goes for dried herbs as well.
* Store in a cool, dry place. If the remedy is used in the bathroom, keep just a small container there and store the rest either in the refrigerator or a cupboard.
* Freezing or refrigeration will extend the life of oils and syrups.

there. It is important to learn which actions each herb has and how it works.

Another thing to consider is whether herbs are associated with a certain organ or body part. This will narrow down your possible choices when approaching an illness or ailment. Here are just a few examples:

OATS nervous system

SOLOMON'S SEAL connective tissues

HAWTHORN AND ROSE heart

MILK THISTLE liver

GOLDENROD kidney

PLEURISY ROOT lining of lungs and chest cavity

If you struggle to classify some herbs, tissues, and illnesses into types and states, that's okay. Even experts don't always agree. As Rosemary Gladstar once told a class I attended, "Put three herbalists in a room, and you'll get three different opinions." The main thing is to trust your knowledge and intuition.

Now you have a lot of tools in your herbal toolbox. You know how to make various herbal concoctions and have an idea of how everything works together. That just leaves the herbs.

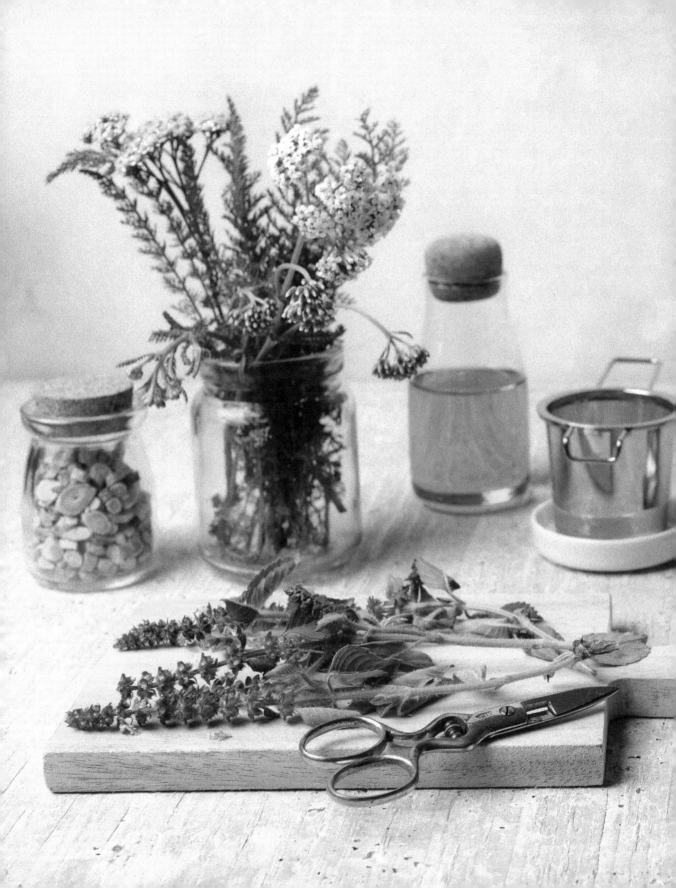

PART II

The 30 Essential Herbs

Finally, it's time to dig into the herbs! I chose the 30 herbs in this section to demonstrate that there are already incredible herbs in your kitchen and everyday life, and also the potential each herb holds for health and healing. Every one of us will wind up having five to 10 favorite herbs. My hope is that of the 30 herbs included here, you will come to love at least five and keep them in your house at all times.

This section features all kinds of recipes, and they are meant to be guidelines; feel free to swap in different herbs depending on your needs and preferences. Learn how to blend herbal teas, make syrups the kids will love, and whip up simple tinctures and elixirs, yummy honeys and vinegars, and salves and massage oils for boo-boos and sore muscles. Knowing how to make these things will empower you to use more natural remedies and take control when it comes to your health and the health of your loved ones.

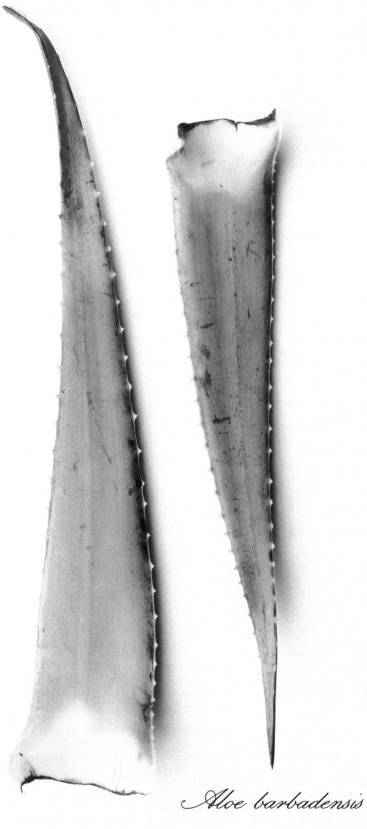

Aloe barbadensis

ALOE

Revered and used medicinally for thousands of years, the succulent beauty aloe is native to India and Africa (including Egypt) and has more than 400 known species. The origin word for aloe is the Arabic *alloeh*, meaning "bitter and shiny substance." *The Egyptian Book of Remedies* from 1500 BC mentions aloe. In the Bible, Nicodemus mixed aloe with myrrh to apply to Christ's body. Later, Alexander the Great fought for it, and Greek physician Dioscorides wrote about it. Such a sought-after plant, yet it turns out that it practically grows itself. Aloe is a welcome houseplant anywhere and freely grows outside in certain climates. Even those who scoff at medicinal herbs have probably used aloe at some point!

ABOUT ALOE

OTHER COMMON NAMES burn plant, medicine plant, sinkle bible (in the Caribbean Islands particularly), plant of immortality

SAFETY CONSIDERATIONS Regular and long-term internal use of aloe can cause chronic diarrhea and at high doses may cause liver damage, so it is strongly discouraged beyond occasional use. Aloe should not be used internally during pregnancy or while breastfeeding. If you use insulin or blood thinners or have hypoglycemia, do not take aloe internally. Some individuals may be allergic to it.

PARTS USED The gel and firm pulp (also known as the fillet, or tuna) inside the leaves; the bitter yellow latex, called aloe juice, or sap that forms between the green skin and the clear gel in mature plants. This yellow juice contains the cathartic, laxative properties. While it can be used internally, commercially made aloe juice is much safer.

ENERGETICS bitter, moisturizing, cool

PROPERTIES Aloe is cathartic, anesthetic, anti-inflammatory, antibacterial, antiviral, emollient, and a laxative.

USES Externally, aloe can heal wounds, burns, skin infections, psoriasis, and eczema. Internally, it's good for digestive issues such as IBS, constipation, and ulcers. You can also gargle aloe juice to help heal gingivitis and ulcers in the mouth.

PREPARATIONS Aloe is difficult to preserve, so the best thing to do is grow it as a houseplant—it's nearly impossible to kill—and peel the leaves as needed at the time of use. You can find aloe gel in most drugstores, and capsules made from aloe are also available. Soaps, creams, and lotions made with aloe are widely available. Aloe juice has the consistency of water and is available in most health food stores.

DOSAGE Internally, the gel can be taken in consultation with a health care provider. Commercially available preparations provide specific dosages. Topically, apply the fresh gel as needed. External use has no unsafe limit.

GROWING TIP Anyone can grow aloe. I've seen the plant be ignored for more than a year (given no water), and revive within days after watering. The only way to kill aloe is to overwater it, so let it dry out. Cut leaves from the bottom to use, as they'll be the oldest and largest. Aloe grows as a perennial in zones 9 and 10, with lance-shaped leaves from the basal rosette reaching several feet tall.

Home treatments

Aloe once saved an island vacation. I snorkeled the entire first day and ended up with a severe sunburn. I cut a three-foot aloe leaf from right outside the room and cut slices from it, laying the fillets directly on my burning skin. That soothing, cool, emollient gel helped immediately, and by morning my skin was no longer red.

I see lots of sports and weight loss drinks out there with aloe as an ingredient. There is currently quite a bit of research on using aloe vera gel (not juice) internally for ulcerative colitis and other serious diseases of the gut. However, until more is known about its liver toxicity and possible carcinogenic properties, I will concur with the Center for Science in the Public Interest and suggest avoiding internal use of aloe vera gel.

ALOE MOUTHWASH

Makes 1 cup
Prep time: 5 minutes

Gargling with aloe is terrific for your
gums and helps prevent gingivitis. It
can also be helpful for sore throats.
You can even give it a try the next
time you can't wait for that cheese
pizza to cool and end up with the roof
of your mouth painfully blistered.
Aloe juice is made by pressing the
entire leaf of the aloe, including the
outer green part. It is much easier to
work with than aloe gel, which can
get sticky. The juice is perfect for
this recipe.

INGREDIENTS

½ cup aloe juice

½ cup water

2 teaspoons baking soda

1 drop spearmint essential oil

1 drop tea tree essential oil

1 drop orange essential oil

SUPPLIES

a 10- or 12-ounce jar

1. Combine all the ingredients in a
   10- or 12-ounce jar and shake
   well to dissolve the baking soda.

2. To use, swish an ounce or so
   of the juice in your mouth for
   30 seconds to a minute. Do not
   swallow.

3. Seal the jar and store in the
   refrigerator.

ALOE HAIR MASK

Makes 1 mask for long hair
or 2 masks for short hair
Prep time: 10 minutes

Aloe has a reputation for working wonders on damaged hair, soothing itchy scalps, and relieving dandruff. It leaves hair smooth and shiny. The oil and milk in this mask increase these actions, and the nettle helps strengthen hair and keep it healthy.

INGREDIENTS

¼ cup aloe gel

¼ cup coconut milk

2 tablespoons powdered nettle

1 tablespoon coconut oil

SUPPLIES

an airtight jar

1. In a microwave-safe bowl, combine all the ingredients and mix until smooth.

2. Warm the mixture in the microwave for 30 seconds (or in a double boiler for about 3 minutes), until the coconut oil is melted.

3. Store in an airtight jar and refrigerate.

4. The mask can be used about once a week. Work it through dry hair and into the scalp and spend a few minutes massaging it in. Cover hair with a shower cap or plastic wrap, then cover with a towel to retain the heat. Let the mask sit for about 30 minutes, then rinse, condition, and admire.

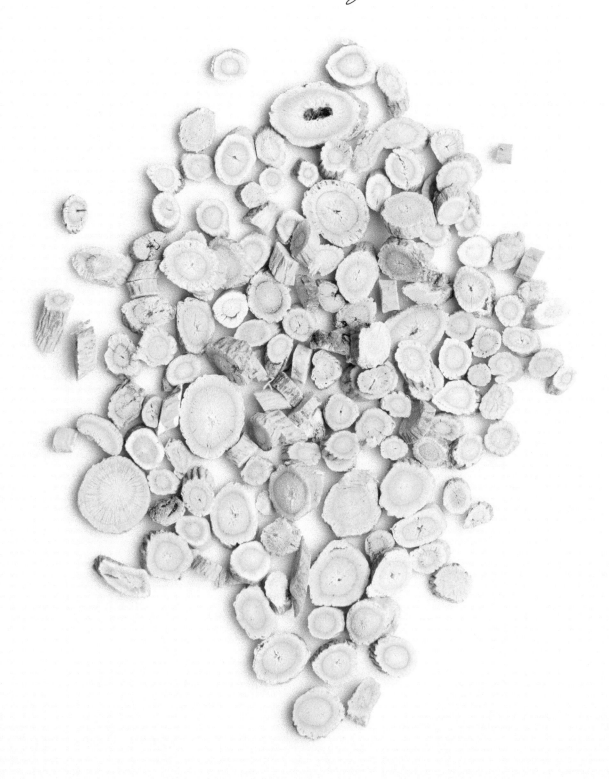

Astragalus membranaceus

ASTRAGALUS

Astragalus is native to China. It's an unassuming vetch with small yellow flowers that ripen into small seedpods resembling tiny beans. It has been used in traditional Chinese medicine for thousands of years and is one of the 50 fundamental herbs used in that tradition. Additionally, it has been used in cooking just as long, making it a perfect example of food as medicine. It has always been considered a healing tonic, but in recent years astragalus has caught the eye of scientific researchers. It shows promise for helping with asthma, high blood pressure, and diabetes, and even slowing the growth of tumors. It's safe to say that use of astragalus will be on the rise in the coming years.

ABOUT ASTRAGALUS

OTHER COMMON NAMES Huangqi (Chinese), milk vetch

SAFETY CONSIDERATIONS Due to its long history of use, astragalus is generally considered safe, but there have not been enough studies done, so do not use during pregnancy or while breastfeeding. Also avoid astragalus if you're using immune suppressant medication or have an autoimmune disease.

PART USED root

ENERGETICS sweet, warm, moisturizing

PROPERTIES Astragalus is a tonic or adaptogenic herb, supporting adrenal function. It is antibacterial, antiviral, diuretic, anti-inflammatory, immune-stimulating, and antiaging. Astragalus contains over 40 saponins, which are soap-like compounds that function to benefit us in many ways, including binding to and removing ammonia, which can be a neurotoxin if not efficiently eliminated. It also contains antioxidants, amino acids, essential fatty acids, and several trace minerals.

USES Astragalus is often used as a preventive or remedy for upper-respiratory illnesses. It stimulates the immune system and also protects the body from the effects of stress. Externally, it soothes and heals the skin. Astragalus is excellent for rebuilding energy and immunity after an illness or when experiencing low energy and strength.

PREPARATIONS Astragalus is available in dried slices and in cut and sifted form. It's also used in decoctions, tinctures, capsules or pills, lotions, and creams. I have seen dried soup mixes of astragalus blended with healing mushrooms and other herbs. There are also several good astragalus teas available.

DOSAGE If using a commercial product, follow the label directions. Take a dropperful (about 25 drops) of astragalus tincture two or three times a day if you feel an illness coming on, or once a day as a daily preventive. During illness, increase your dosage to a strong decoction or tincture two or three times a day, or take capsules twice daily. Broth made with astragalus root is especially healing.

GROWING TIP Astragalus is very easy to grow as a perennial in zones 6 through 9. The vetches can get aggressive, so find a spacious spot where it can spread. You can harvest the roots for use in the fourth year. Dig the outer roots, leaving the center to grow. Clean well, slice, and dry.

Home treatments

Astragalus is good to use after a severe illness. It supports healing and helps strength and vitality return. As an adaptogen and immune stimulant, it is also nourishing and slowly and gently builds us back up. There are several easy ways to incorporate this warming and moistening herb into your days. You can cook the slices into most soups or stews, or sprinkle the shredded root over rice, pasta, or potatoes while they cook. Keep some in the kitchen, and you'll use it more often. The tea is very pleasant tasting and blends well with elderflower and holy basil.

It is well known that stress, whether physical or emotional, wreaks havoc on our organs, manifesting in an inability to fight off any attack. This makes us susceptible to any germ that comes our way. The immune system–supporting and tonic properties of astragalus keep illness and the effects of stress at bay. In my household, we very rarely get sick. As part of our preventive winter herbal arsenal, we add astragalus slices to soups and teas so that we have some almost every day.

TONIC SOUP

Serves 8
Prep time: 90 minutes
(30 minutes active)

Warming and delicious, this soup gives immunity a boost. It freezes well, so it's easy to keep on hand through the winter. There's nothing like soup to keep the chills away.

INGREDIENTS

8 cups broth (beef, chicken, or vegetable)

1 tablespoon olive oil

1 onion, diced

4 to 8 cloves garlic, minced

1 (1-inch) piece fresh gingerroot, peeled and finely chopped

1 cup sliced carrots

1 cup fresh burdock root (sold in stores as gobo) or sweet potatoes, chopped into bite-size pieces

2 slices astragalus root

1 cup shiitake mushrooms (fresh or reconstituted), sliced

3 cups kale or collard greens, chopped into ½-inch pieces

SUPPLIES

a large pot and a skillet

1. In a large pot over high heat, bring the broth to a boil.

2. Meanwhile, heat the olive oil in a skillet over medium heat and add the onion, garlic, and ginger. Reduce the heat to low and sauté until soft and fragrant.

3. Add the contents of the skillet to the broth in the pot, along with the carrots, burdock root, astragalus root, and mushrooms.

4. Simmer, covered, over low heat for 50 minutes.

5. Add the greens and simmer for 10 more minutes.

6. Remove the astragalus with a fork or tongs before serving.

7. Refrigerate leftovers.

IMMUNITY BALLS

Makes 48 (1-inch) balls
Prep time: 1 hour

This recipe is a take on Rosemary Gladstar's Zoom Balls, but in this version we use herbs to stimulate and support the immune system. You can substitute almost any ingredient to your taste preferences or needs. For instance, you can use sunflower seed butter if nuts are a problem. Eat a couple of these a day during flu season for a tasty, nutritious, immunity-boosting snack.

INGREDIENTS

1 cup cashew, almond, or peanut butter

½ cup honey or blackstrap molasses

¼ cup astragalus powder

¼ cup calendula powder

¼ cup echinacea powder

¼ cup holy basil powder

½ cup cocoa powder, divided (optional)

1 tablespoon ground ginger

1 tablespoon ground cardamom

1 tablespoon ground cinnamon

½ cup shredded coconut (optional)

SUPPLIES

an airtight container

1. In a bowl, using a large spoon, mix together the nut butter with the honey.

2. Gradually add the astragalus, calendula, echinacea, and holy basil powders; ¼ cup cocoa (if using); and the ginger, cardamom, and cinnamon to the mixture to form a stiff dough.

3. Roll into bite-size balls. If desired, roll them in the remaining ¼ cup cocoa and/or the shredded coconut.

4. Store the balls in an airtight container at room temperature or in the refrigerator.

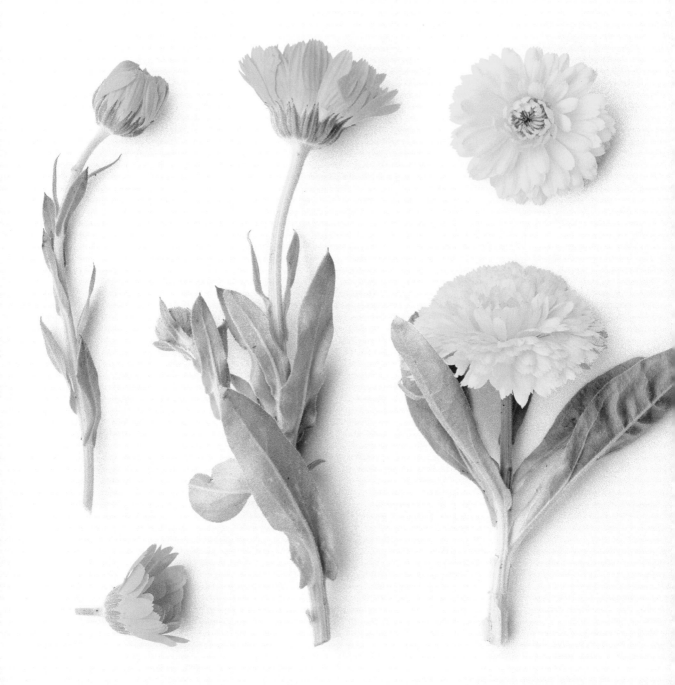

Calendula officinalis

CALENDULA

Calendula has been worn, eaten, and used for healing for centuries. In ancient Roman times, it was noted that calendula flowers opened to the sun and closed at night, and were always in bloom on the first day of each month of the Roman calendar, or on each full moon. The herb's name is related to the passage of time, and the bright yellow and orange blooms look just like the sun. Calendula is part of many traditional rituals. It's still used today in Día de Los Muertos celebrations, and Hindu altars are often decorated with the bright flowers. The Aztecs and other ancient Central and South American peoples revered the little sun plant. Calendula is a medicinal herb. Whenever the word *officinalis* (or *officinale*) appears in a Latin plant name, it denotes use in medicine and herbalism.

ABOUT CALENDULA

OTHER COMMON NAMES pot marigold, poor man's saffron, ruddles, common marigold, calendule, Mary's gold, Mary bud, English garden marigold, Scotch marigold, or poet's marigold

SAFETY CONSIDERATIONS Those allergic to plants in the aster family should avoid calendula. Women in early pregnancy should avoid internal use. Otherwise, the herb is considered quite safe for both internal and external use.

PARTS USED Flowers and leaves, which contain a sticky resin that is herbal gold, indicating the powerful healing properties held within the plant.

ENERGETICS bitter, warm, drying

PROPERTIES The plant has many amazing and valuable qualities. Because it is antiviral, anti-inflammatory, antibacterial, styptic, vulnerary, antispasmodic, and astringent, it was found to be useful on the battlefields during the Civil War. It is still a favorite herb for taking care of injuries and illness. Calendula's high level of carotenoids helps fight free radicals, which can cause aging and disease.

USES Calendula is commonly used for skin issues and wounds. It's even gentle enough to use in products for babies, such as diaper cream or scalp oil for cradle cap. It can make a huge difference on foot or leg ulcers, particularly when combined with comfrey. Used internally, it helps mucus membranes heal, so it's quite useful for digestive and gastrointestinal problems. You can use calendula as a gargle or rinse for the gums and throat. Calendula tea has a history of working as an eyewash to relieve symptoms of pink eye. Personally, I like to make a very wet, warm tea compress for the eyes.

PREPARATIONS You can find (or make) calendula oil, salves, teas, tinctures, gels, lotions, creams, poultices, compresses, and soaps. There are also lots of food uses.

DOSAGE As with most of the plants that are also used as food, dosage of calendula isn't critical; it depends almost entirely on the issue being addressed.

GROWING TIP Calendula is very easy to grow; I simply scatter the seeds in the spring. It's best to cover them with ½ inch of dirt after all danger of frost has passed. They will germinate quickly and bloom from July until frost. After drying, the seeds look like small worms among the petals. Don't toss them—save them to plant next spring.

Home treatments

Calendula tea is good as a single or part of a blend (with lemon balm, elderberry, holy basil, and rose) to boost the immune system. Being antispasmodic, the warm tea has been known to calm abdominal or menstrual cramps.

Calendula is great for wounds that aren't healing. The drying energy specifically helps weepy wounds or rashes, helping clear them up. During our shop days, a woman with an ulcer on her ankle the size of a half-dollar came in and said her prescriptions weren't helping. She was in tears. We recommended a salve of calendula and goldenseal. She came in a week later for more, and the ulcer was only half as big. She'd used it three times a day, cleaning the wound every evening.

CALENDULA SUNSHINE BATH SOAK

Makes 12 bath soaks
Prep time: 15 minutes

This is a rejuvenating and soothing bath that feels incredible after too much time in the sun or garden. The magnesium in Epsom salts is great for overworked muscles. With the addition of some other ingredients, you'll step out of the bath a new person. The scents and healing properties of the herbs along with the pure relaxation of a warm bath combine to heal scratches, bug bites, wind, or sunburn.

INGREDIENTS

1 cup calendula flowers, chopped

1 cup comfrey leaves

½ cup yarrow

¼ cup elderflowers

3 tablespoons lavender

20 drops lemon essential oil

3 cups Epsom salts

SUPPLIES

a large jar or plastic container

a muslin bag or washcloth

1. Combine all the botanicals in a bowl or large plastic bag.

2. In a separate bowl, combine the essential oil and Epsom salts and mix.

3. Mix everything together and place in a large, wide-mouthed jar. If you're keeping it near the tub, a (recycled) plastic jar is probably safest.

4. To use, place ½ cup of the soak in a muslin bag or into a washcloth and tie securely. Heat a quart of water on the stove and steep the bath soak in it for 10 to 15 minutes.

5. Pour the hot liquid into the bath. Soak.

ALL-PURPOSE CALENDULA SALVE

Makes 8 to 10 ounces
Prep time: 15 minutes after calendula oil is infused (infusion time depends on method used)

This salve comes in handy all year. From small boo-boos and skeeter bites to burns, cuts, chapped hands, and bruises, it soothes everything. I like to use it on days I forget to put moisturizer on my face, too.

INGREDIENTS

1 cup fresh (or ½ cup dried) calendula flowers

1½ cups olive oil

1 to 1½ ounces beeswax (see Tip)

20 drops lavender essential oil (optional)

20 drops tea tree essential oil (optional)

SUPPLIES

a few small jars

TIP If you have 8 ounces of oil after straining, use 1 ounce of beeswax. If you have more than 8 ounces, use 1½ ounces of the beeswax.

1. Use whatever method you prefer to infuse the calendula into the oil (see page 16).

2. Strain (a strainer lined with cloth is best) the oil well, squeezing as much oil from the flowers as possible. The goal is to have at least 8 ounces of the oil.

3. In a pot, gently heat the oil with the beeswax until the wax is liquefied. Stir the mixture well to be sure all the wax is incorporated.

4. If including the essential oils, add them to the mixture.

5. Pour the salve into jars. When it has hardened and cooled, place lids on the jars and store in a cool place.

6. To use, apply a thin layer of salve to the skin and gently massage it in.

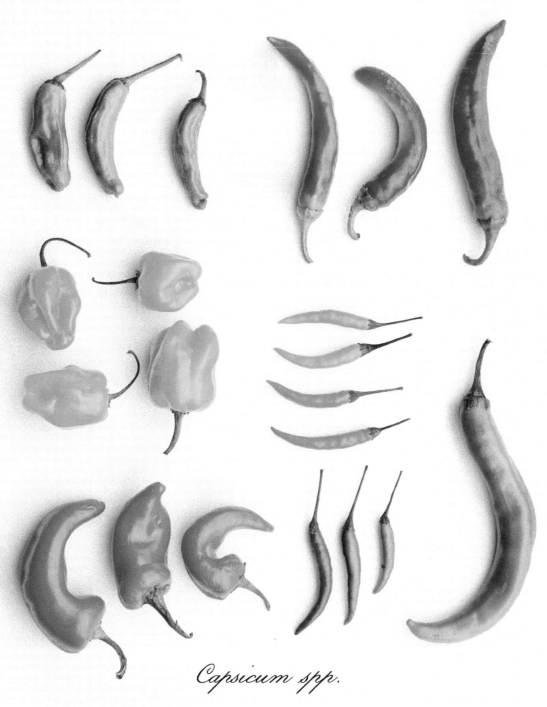

Capsicum spp.

Capsicum annuum, Capsicum frutescens, Capsicum chinense,
Capsicum pubescens, Capsicum baccatum

CAPSICUM

All peppers except sweet bell peppers contain capsicum. Peppers are from the nightshade family, along with tomatoes, potatoes, and eggplants. Hot, spicy peppers have been cultivated in Mexico, Central America, and South America for at least 3,000 years, with some sources going back 7,000 years. Dishes from Jamaica, India, various African countries, China, Korea, Louisiana, Mexico, and Central and South America all include hot peppers and have been making their way to the United States and parts of Europe in the last century. As a child, I had zero contact with hot foods, and I was nearly 30 when I first found them to be delicious. Capsicum is not just a flavorful, enlivening spice for foods. It also has plenty of benefits for health and comfort, not the least of which is its high content of carotenoids and vitamins C and E.

ABOUT CAPSICUM

OTHER COMMON NAMES red pepper, chile, cayenne, hot pepper

SAFETY CONSIDERATIONS Avoid external use on children under 2 years of age. Do not apply to broken skin or use near the eyes or mucus membranes. Internal overdose can cause nausea, vomiting, abdominal pain, and burning diarrhea.

PARTS USED Fruit, whole pepper. Many people believe that the seeds are the hottest part, but it is actually the surrounding tissue that holds and clings to the seeds.

ENERGETICS warming

PROPERTIES Capsicum has so much to offer. It is antifungal, antimicrobial, carminative, diaphoretic, expectorant, immune-stimulating, and styptic, and it gets the metabolism moving. The active ingredient, an irritant alkaloid called capsaicin, encourages circulation and thins blood. Capsicum stimulates gastric juices and saliva to improve digestion. It also stimulates perspiration, helping cool a fever.

USES For years people with digestive issues were told to avoid spicy foods and stick to bland diets, but capsicum aids in digestion and helps problems, including upset stomach, intestinal gas, stomach pain, diarrhea, and cramps.

Some evidence suggests it may help with diabetes and weight management, as well as headaches, blood pressure regulation, and heart disease.

Externally, a salve, gel, lotion, or patch on the skin can bring relief to lingering pain post-shingles, the joint pains of osteoarthritis, rheumatoid arthritis, and fibromyalgia, as well as everyday muscle and joint aches.

PREPARATIONS You can find or make capsicum topical salves, gels, lotions, and patches. For internal use, capsules, vinegar, or tinctures work well. The herb is also a terrific food ingredient or seasoning.

DOSAGE On commercial products, follow the dose instructions. External preparations can be used three or four times a day. Discontinue if a rash develops. Internally, take as tolerated.

GROWING TIP Peppers are easy to grow by seed. The plants are also becoming popular at nurseries and heirloom herb festivals. Be sure to keep sweet and hot peppers as far apart as possible because they will cross-pollinate, and the heat always wins.

Peppers appear on the plant green, turn yellow, then turn orange, ripening to red. Some are purple or brown.

Home treatments

The Cayenne Salve (page 59) is a lifesaver for me in winter. Here in Pennsylvania, the term "bone-chilling" means that my knees and shoulders ache in the cold season. I apply cayenne salve morning and night to get blood to the area and knock out the pain.

Note that this is a warming and stimulating herb. Capsicum stimulates, moves, and flushes things around and out. If you've ever watched a hot pepper-eating contest, you've seen how saliva, tears, perspiration, and mucus all flow freely. Not the most pleasant sight! Health-wise, an example of this is a case of blocked sinuses—those times when it feels like you're living with a fishbowl over your head. As soon as you eat some spicy food with cayenne, it warms you up, stimulates perspiration and mucus production, and flushes out that blockage.

HOT SAUCE

Makes about 2 cups
Prep time: 90 minutes
(45 minutes active)

Adding hot and spicy capsicum to meals is a good way to reap the medicinal benefits of peppers. Having a bottle of this hot sauce on hand makes it easy to season and spice up your meals. It packs a big punch in both flavor and healing. Word to the wise: Wear gloves while preparing this, as it is very hard to get all the oil off your hands.

INGREDIENTS

1½ cups rice vinegar

2 dozen hot red peppers (I like a mixture of whatever is available), coarsely chopped

½ medium red bell pepper, coarsely chopped

1 medium onion, diced

5 garlic cloves, chopped

½ teaspoon salt

SUPPLIES

rubber gloves

a stick blender

a few bottles or jars

1. Pour the rice vinegar into a medium pot. Add all the peppers, the onion, garlic, and salt.

2. Bring to a boil, then simmer for about 10 minutes, until the peppers are soft.

3. Using an immersion blender, whirl the mixture into a liquid.

4. Simmer uncovered to reduce for 5 minutes.

5. Pour the hot sauce into bottles. Store at room temperature or refrigerate.

CAYENNE SALVE

Makes 12 to 14 ounces
Prep time: 4½ to 6½ hours (10 min-utes prep, 4 to 6 hours to infuse, 10 minutes to create salve)

The heat from the peppers and the ginger in this salve promote circula-tion to speed healing while relieving pain. The peppermint oil is cooling and analgesic, making the combina-tion very effective.

INGREDIENTS

2 cups olive oil

½ cup dried hot peppers

1 tablespoon grated fresh ginger

2 ounces beeswax

1 teaspoon peppermint essential oil

SUPPLIES

a slow cooker

assorted jars

1. In a slow cooker on low, infuse the olive oil with the peppers and ginger for 4 to 6 hours.

2. Strain and pour into a glass measuring cup or other container with a pouring lip. While the oil is still hot, stir in the beeswax until it melts.

3. Add the essential oil just before pouring the salve into jars.

4. To use, apply cooled salve directly to the skin using an ice pop stick or the back of a spoon (this keeps bacteria from being introduced into the jar).

TIP It's easiest to put peppers and ginger into a muslin bag and submerge in the oil while infusing. Remove the whole bag when finished.

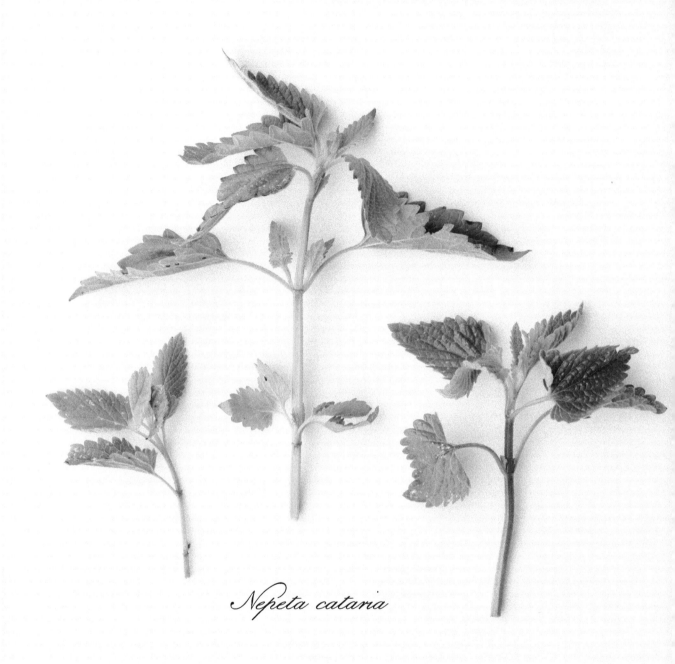

Nepeta cataria

CATNIP

Catnip is often relegated to the feline family, but we shouldn't be so quick to write it off for humans. As with most plants waving around out there in the sunshine, catnip has some gifts to offer us as well.

I consider catnip and catmint to be two different plants, but in most literature the two are considered to be the same. Catnip is the wild and scruffy wayside herb that grows chest high with thick spikes of tiny white flowers. Catmint, on the other hand, is much more refined, with small leaves and pretty blue flower spikes; it grows to a height of two to three feet. They are both lovely, fragrant, and at the ready to assist with several maladies.

ABOUT CATNIP

OTHER COMMON NAMES catmint, catswort, catnep, field balm

SAFETY CONSIDERATIONS Avoid catnip while pregnant or if you have kidney or liver issues.

PARTS USED Leaves and flowers, particularly while in bloom if you're looking for insect repellent properties.

ENERGETICS cool, dry, slightly bitter

PROPERTIES Catnip has a lot going for it, being antispasmodic, diaphoretic (thereby reducing fevers), relaxing and sedative, immune-stimulating, mildly anesthetic, and antibiotic. It contains antioxidants, flavonoids, vitamins C and E, and minerals like chromium, iron, manganese, potassium, and selenium. Some individuals say that catnip is a psychedelic intoxicant when smoked, but there's no research to support this. Nepetalactone is the constituent responsible for catnip's reactions, but it is also a repellent for (oddly) cats, small rodents, and several insects. Several studies from the turn of the century show that catnip essential oil is more effective than DEET against mosquitoes.

USES Catnip is occasionally used in place of chamomile because it has similar relaxing, calming, and stomach-soothing properties. It is very helpful for colds, the flu, cramps, colic or indigestion, headaches, insomnia, and restlessness. The anti-inflammatory properties make it effective for arthritis, and poultices soothe hemorrhoids, hives, and bug bites. The tea may also help new mothers relax to nurse their babies.

PREPARATIONS Catnip can be found dried and as teas, tinctures, salves, capsules, and essential oils.

DOSAGE It is safe to use the tea, tincture, and capsules up to three times a day. If using the maximum amounts each day, give your body a few days off after a week or so (this method is known as "pulsing") before using again. Use salve as needed. Be sure the essential oil is properly diluted before you use. Leaves of the fresh plant rubbed onto the skin will also work to repel mosquitoes.

HARVESTING TIP It's worthwhile to gather some wild blooming catnip during the summer. It takes quite a bit of the fresh herb to dry down to a few ounces.

Home treatments

Catnip is a brilliant remedy for the restlessness that keeps kids (and adults) from settling down to sleep. I always prefer a tea as a relaxing remedy for its warmth, and because it encourages me to stop and sip it. Sometimes I could get my child to have a tea party, but when it wasn't possible to reason with her (you know how cranky tired kids can be), tinctures were great. They relaxed her and settled any tummy troubles.

Catnip tea is perfect for colds and the flu. It blends well with other herbs and makes a good base herb, since it has a pleasant, mildly minty flavor. It can help dry up drippy colds and get a sweat going to break a fever. Mixed with boneset and elderberry, catnip in tea or tinctures contains properties that boost the immune system, calm cramping, relieve pain, and enable rest during the flu. If there's vomiting, a tincture can be easier to keep down than cups of tea.

CATNIP AND ROSE GERANIUM BUG REPELLING SPRAY

Makes about 1 quart
Prep time: 15 minutes plus 2 weeks to steep

The botanicals in this natural bug spray are as effective as harsh chemicals, without the dangerous side effects. In recent years, ticks and mosquitoes have been found to carry new diseases, so avoiding their bites is more important than ever.

FOR THE ALCOHOL

2 cups blooming fresh catnip, finely chopped

1 cup fresh rose geranium, finely chopped

1 cup lemongrass, chopped

½ cup lavender

1 quart 80- or 100-proof vodka

FOR THE OIL

1 cup olive oil

2 tablespoons blooming fresh catnip, chopped

2 tablespoons fresh rose geranium, chopped

2 tablespoons lemongrass

2 tablespoons lavender

30 drops lemon eucalyptus essential oil

SUPPLIES

a jar

some spray bottles

TO MAKE THE ALCOHOL

1. Place the botanicals in a jar and cover with the vodka.

2. Let steep at room temperature for 2 weeks. Strain and return the liquid to the jar.

TO MAKE THE OIL

1. In a baking dish, combine the oil, catnip, rose geranium, lemongrass, and lavender. Put in the oven at the lowest setting (180°F to 200°F, generally labeled "warm") for 2 hours.

2. Strain the oil into a large measuring cup.

TO MAKE THE SPRAY

1. Add the alcohol to the measuring cup along with the essential oil and mix.

2. Pour into spray bottles.

3. To use, spray directly onto skin. Shake vigorously between uses to be sure the alcohol and oil combine for a longer-lasting repellent.

RELAXING CATNIP TEA BLEND

Makes enough for 12 cups
Prep time: 15 minutes

The ingredients in this blend work together to relax and soothe. They make a pretty blend, too. I like to make sure the experience of the tea complements the desired effect. Use a beautiful cup; sit in a favorite chair—whatever makes you feel pampered and calm. This enhances the herbal properties, and besides, you deserve it.

INGREDIENTS

¼ cup dried catnip

3 tablespoons dried lemon balm
(see Note)

3 tablespoons dried chamomile

1 tablespoon dried rose petals

SUPPLIES

an 8-ounce jar

1. In an 8-ounce jar (a half-pint Mason jar is perfect), blend all the herbs together well.

2. In a tea kettle, put water on to just reach a boil.

3. To make 1 cup of tea, put 2 teaspoons of the tea blend in a mug and pour in 8 ounces (1 cup) of the hot water.

4. Cover and let steep for 5 to 10 minutes.

5. Store the leftover tea blend in the sealed jar at room temperature.

NOTE Those on thyroid medication should check with their doctor before using lemon balm.

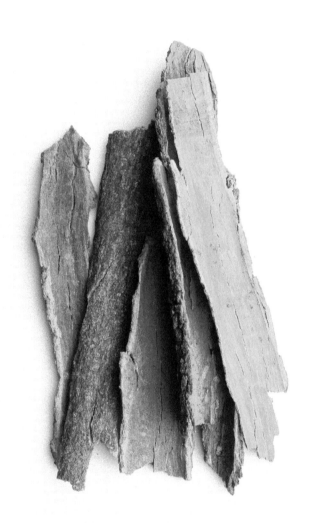

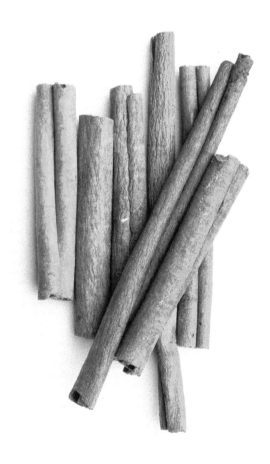

Cinnamomum verum

AND THE MORE COMMON *Cinnamomum aromaticum (cassia)*

CINNAMON

Cinnamon is one of the most commonly used culinary spices. You can find it in all types of baked goods and desserts, and it flavors everything from breakfast dishes to soup to nuts. Most of the cinnamon commercially available is the *aromaticum* variety, also known as cassia, coming from China and parts of Southeast Asia. The *verum* variety is preferred—it has a more delicate flavor and is favored for medicinal use because it contains less coumarin, which thins the blood. It is thinner than cassia, almost papery, and tan. Cassia is one thick reddish-brown layer of curled bark. However, *verum* can be difficult to find and is more expensive.

ABOUT CINNAMON

OTHER COMMON NAMES cannelle, canela, Laurus cinnamomum, dalchini

SAFETY CONSIDERATIONS The coumarin in cassia is a blood thinner, so it is not recommended for individuals on blood-thinner medication. When used in large quantities, such as the daily dosage for medicinal purposes, coumarin is a liver and kidney toxin. Cinnamon essential oil is a skin irritant and somewhat caustic. Always dilute cinnamon essential oil, and opt for leaf oil rather than bark oil.

PARTS USED inner bark, leaves

ENERGETICS hot, dry, pungent, sweet, warming

PROPERTIES Cinnamon is anti-inflammatory, and is thought to have more antioxidants than almost any other food in the world. It has antibacterial, antifungal, antiviral properties that combine to boost immunity. It is also antiseptic, astringent, carminative, and a stimulant, and contains calcium and tons of manganese.

USES Cinnamon helps stop vomiting, relieves flatulence, and is useful in getting rid of diarrhea. Some medical doctors are now encouraging their patients to consume cinnamon each day to reduce blood sugar, blood pressure, and cholesterol levels. You can use cinnamon tea for nausea or apply it externally for fungus. Cinnamon essential oil is a potent antibacterial and antifungal ointment.

PREPARATIONS Cinnamon can be found or made as teas, capsules, or essential oils. The easiest usage is as a food ingredient (even cinnamon buns are medicinal!), and it comes in sticks or powder.

DOSAGE If using *verum,* the daily dosage is ½ to 1 teaspoon, one to three capsules, or one to three cups of tea. If using cassia, cut these doses in half given the higher coumarin content. Be wary of commercial labels—many suppliers use the cheaper cassia without explicitly saying so.

COOKING TIP The flavor of freshly grated cinnamon is so much better than the stuff that comes in the jars. I like to grate it at home with my Microplane grater. It takes a bit of work, but it's worth it. Add to some fresh apples for homemade applesauce—yum!

Home treatments

Many doctors are now aware of cinnamon's positive effects on blood sugar, cholesterol, sensitivity to insulin, brain activity, allergies, and neurological function in diseases like Alzheimer's and Parkinson's, and they recommend it to their patients. Because the therapeutic amount of *verum* cinnamon is generally recognized as safe, there is no reason not to try it if you have a condition that might be improved.

Drinking a cup of cinnamon tea every day is a pleasant way to stimulate and boost the immune system, and in winter it is a comforting morning or afternoon warm-up. To make cinnamon tea, heat water in a kettle and pour it into a cup with a stick of cinnamon. Let steep for 8 to 10 minutes. Remove the cinnamon, which will have probably uncurled and flattened. It will curl up again as it dries, and you can keep it for many more cups. Add honey and enjoy.

SPICY CHAI

Makes 4 cups
Prep time: 15 minutes

It is well worth gathering all the delicious spices for this sweet, warm, and rich beverage. Each one is packed with health benefits and healing powers, and the combination packs a big flavor punch. This is the perfect hot drink for the cooler months.

INGREDIENTS

3 slices fresh ginger

6 cloves

1 (3-inch) cinnamon stick, broken into small pieces

1 tablespoon dried holy basil

½ teaspoon coriander seeds

3 black peppercorns

3 cardamom pods

½ teaspoon fennel seeds

3 tea bags black tea

3 cups cold water

6 to 8 tablespoons half-and-half

2 tablespoons honey

SUPPLIES

a saucepan

Gently warm all the ingredients in a saucepan, covered, for 10 to 15 minutes. Do not let the mixture boil. Using a strainer, strain the warm chai into a teapot. Serve.

TIP You can premix all the spices (except for the fresh ginger) in muslin bags to use for future brews.

CINNAMON HONEY

Makes 12 ounces
Prep time: 10 minutes

All of the medicinal properties of cinnamon are at your fingertips with this delicious and versatile honey "medicine." Spread it on buttered toast, add it to green tea, toss a spoonful into a meat dish, or just eat it by the spoonful. The honey complements the cinnamon, and has lots of health benefits on its own.

INGREDIENTS

1 cup local raw organic honey

½ cup ground (fresh, if possible) *verum* cinnamon

SUPPLIES

a jar or two for storing

1. Pour the honey into a bowl. If it seems too thick, you can heat it a little bit: Simply place the container of honey in a bowl of hot water, or microwave in 30-second increments until it thins.

2. Carefully add the cinnamon a little at a time, stirring well.

3. Spoon the flavored honey into a jar or two.

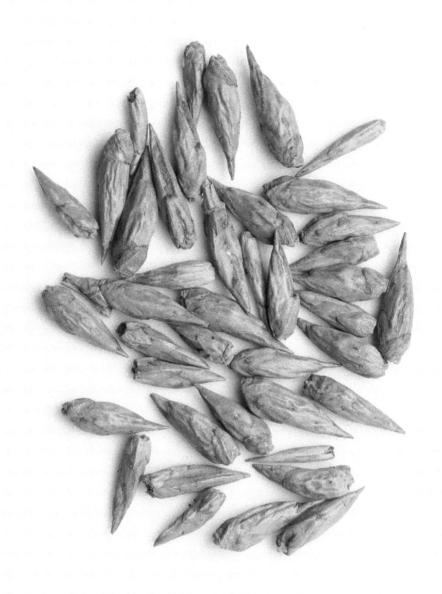

Populus spp.

P. balsamifera, P. deltoides, P. angustifolia, P. trichocarpa, P. candicans

COTTONWOOD OR BALSAM POPLAR

There are about 35 species of poplar throughout the U.S. and Canada. Like its close relative willow, poplar is of the Salicaceae family, which means it has the pain-relieving compound salicin, a compound that is converted into the natural form of aspirin, salicylic acid in the liver. Some poplars are known as cottonwoods because of the way their seeds disperse into wild and woolly drifts of white fluff. Their wood is lightweight and soft, which may also influence the name. Their range skips over Pennsylvania, and they aren't native where I live, so the first time I saw the "snow" phenomenon, we stopped the car and stood among the drifts, watching in wonder as the light breeze cornered the fluff against walls and curbing. Cottonwoods and balsam poplars have an amazing healing resin. Some historically traditional First Nation uses include applying the boiled bark to wounds and using the resin as glue to waterproof canoes.

ABOUT COTTONWOOD OR BALSAM POPLAR

OTHER COMMON NAMES balm of Gilead, poplar, black cottonwood, snow in summer, the people's tree

SAFETY CONSIDERATIONS People allergic to aspirin should not use.

PARTS USED Most often the buds are used and occasionally the leaves and bark. The catkins are an edible source of vitamin C.

ENERGETICS cool, dry, astringent, bitter

PROPERTIES These trees offer a lot of healing. They are analgesic, antiinflammatory, antibacterial, antimicrobial, and antiseptic, with aromatics. They're also expectorant, astringent, and diuretic, and they thin the blood and reduce fevers.

Inner bark used as tea or decoction internally is tonic and alterative, as well as being a stimulating, cathartic, and diuretic herb, depending upon the amount used.

USES Best known for relieving muscle aches and pains, bruises, swollen joints, and arthritis pain, but there is so much more. Due to the strong healing properties, it is applied to eczema, cuts, rashes, burns, psoriasis, insect bites and stings, sunburn, athlete's foot, dry and scaly skin, chapped hands or cheeks, and diaper rash. It cools the heat and inflammation of wounds and rashes. Aromatics of the resin make it valuable for insomnia, and a tea is used as a gargle for sore throat. It can be used effectively both as a decoction and a chest rub for clearing loose, damp upper-respiratory gunk and coughs. Several herbalists have reported that the resinous oil keeps base oils (like olive, coconut, shea, etc.) from going rancid, but it has never lasted me long enough to find out.

PREPARATIONS The resin is used in oils, salves, teas, decoctions, lip balms, tinctures, poultices, and (rarely) essential oil. Dried buds are available, but their usefulness is questionable. Fresh buds are very difficult to find for sale, but the oil is sometimes available.

DOSAGE FOR LISTED PREPARATIONS External preparations can be used as needed. Internally, decoctions or tinctures may be taken several times daily.

HARVESTING TIPS Oil hands well before beginning harvest so resin sticks less—take along high-proof alcohol to finish hand cleanup. Most people harvest into bags, but consider putting cottonwood or balsam poplar directly into mason jars to be covered later with oil or alcohol. Freeze some whole for decoctions later, and gather some inner bark from fallen branches.

Home treatments

The cool and dry energetics of cottonwood and poplar bring many instances to mind where they would be the perfect remedy.

Hot, weepy rashes or swollen bug bites call out for cottonwood. Aromatically, it is vaguely reminiscent of Peru balsam but doesn't have the extreme sensitizing potential. It seems to have similar skin-soothing and healing properties. A balm made for diaper rash with infused oils of the resin, calendula, and plantain is a quick fix.

Internally, those cooling and drying energetics, along with all the strong healing and protective properties, make it a superior respiratory helper. As a stimulating expectorant, it moves heavy, stagnant mucus up and out. A tincture made with a half jar of buds that have been left out for 24 to 48 hours and filled to the top with 75 percent (151-proof) or 95 percent (190-proof) alcohol for at least two weeks is the most effective means, and also helps with achiness.

COTTONWOOD DECOCTION

Makes 2 cups
Prep time: 1 hour

This recipe can be multiplied to make ahead and freeze into ice cubes. It will come in handy during the year as a medicinal tea taken internally for many of the ailments listed, as a wash or compress to use on skin problems where a salve or oil would be contra-indicated, or as both a tea and wash at once. When it is handy, it's surprising how often you'll pull a few cubes from the freezer and silently thank yourself for planning ahead.

INGREDIENTS

4 cups water

3 tablespoons fresh or frozen cottonwood buds

1 tablespoon dried peppermint

2 teaspoons chopped fresh turmeric or ginger (or heaping ½ teaspoon dried)

Good-quality honey, for sweetening

SUPPLIES

a saucepan

1. In a saucepan over high heat, combine the water, cottonwood buds, peppermint, and turmeric and bring to a boil.

2. Reduce the heat to low and simmer until the liquid is reduced by half.

3. Strain well.

4. Use immediately, sweetened with honey to taste, or freeze for later use.

COTTONWOOD HERBAL LINIMENT

Makes 3 ½ cups
Prep time: 15 minutes,
plus 2 weeks to steep

When creating this liniment, the intention was for the alcohol-based formula to be applicable both internally and externally. This can also be made into an oil-based liniment, which is more penetrating and stays on the skin longer. The oil can easily be made into a salve with the addition of a little beeswax.

INGREDIENTS

1 cup cottonwood

½ cup calendula

½ cup St John's wort

¼ cup peppermint

1 quart 151-proof alcohol or olive oil

SUPPLIES

jars and bottles for storing

ALCOHOL-BASED

Place all the herbs in a jar and cover with alcohol. Seal with a lid and shake a couple of times a day for 2 weeks to loosen and release all the resin. Strain and bottle. Use internally like a tincture.

OIL-BASED

Place all the herbs in a jar and cover with oil. Leave a couple inches of headspace. Affix a lid and place in a warm place for at least 2 weeks. Strain and bottle.

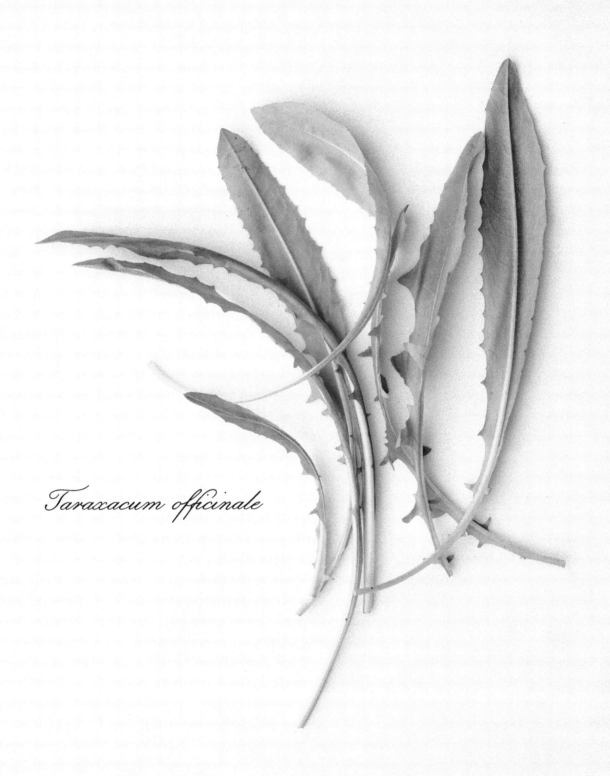

Taraxacum officinale

DANDELION

This is often the first herb that people forage after they figure out it's that plant out there growing everywhere in their yard. Luckily, we will probably never endanger dandelion, even though we've spent the last 70 years trying to spray it into oblivion—dandelion is almost insolent about it. Today, you can even find it at the farmers' market. The greens are delectable, easy to find, and have immense health benefits.

ABOUT DANDELION

OTHER COMMON NAMES lion's tooth, dent de lion

SAFETY CONSIDERATIONS Dandelion is generally recognized as safe.

PARTS USED all parts of the plant except the seeds

ENERGETICS cool, bitter, dry, moisturizing

PROPERTIES Dandelion is an outstanding tonic, pain reliever, decongestant, digestive, diuretic, immune-stimulant, and laxative. It is astringent and assists breastfeeding mothers in lactation. It is rich in vitamins A, C, and E, and calcium. Dandelion wakes us up and gets us moving. The leaves are antioxidant and work to break fevers, normalize blood pressure, restore balance, and speed wound healing. The roots are also antibacterial, antifungal, and anti-inflammatory, and protect the liver and alleviate rheumatism. The roots have the ability to clear obstructions and open ducts of body fluids and secretions. The flowers are pain-relieving and emollient, support liver function, and help wounds heal. The sap is antifungal and pain-relieving.

USES Dandelion helps a wide array of skin issues, such as acne, dullness, eczema, bruising, and rashes, by supporting the liver. It also supports healthy functioning of the kidneys, spleen, and gallbladder, and is thought to be a consistently reliable detoxifying herb. It is often used to stimulate the appetite, support digestion, and relieve excess gas or constipation. The bitter properties increase bile production, in turn helping balance blood sugar levels. Dandelion's diuretic properties make it an excellent choice for the entire urinary system, including the kidneys and bladder, cleansing and tonifying without being too drying. Dandelion is also helpful for symptoms of PMS, removing excess water from the system, relieving pain, and cooling irritability. The diuretic, pain-relieving, and detoxifying abilities also help with gout and edema.

PREPARATIONS You can find or make dandelion teas, tinctures, vinegars, salves, and capsules.

DOSAGE It's safe to use several cups of tea or doses of tincture or capsules daily.

GROWING TIP You may like the bitter flavor of dandelion, but you can shade them in order to "blanch" them, which produces a milder flavor. A relative of mine kept a wooden frame around a patch of dandelions, with boards on top to shield it from the sun. The plants stayed pale and mild into early summer.

Home treatments

Dried dandelion leaves work wonders as a diuretic for water retention. You can make tea with the dried leaves, or it's even easier to make a fresh tincture. Either works. You can also sprinkle dried dandelion leaves into meals, soups, and sauces. Dandelion came to the rescue in one such case for a man with a completely shot liver, meaning it was critical for him to keep all of his mineral and electrolyte levels in balance. He retained huge amounts of water, so we had to find a diuretic that did not deplete his potassium. I powdered dry dandelion leaves and put them in his food daily, with wonderful results.

As a great daily tonic, try dandelion root as a substitute. The roots dry well and get very hard. Before drying them, chop them into small pieces. Roast them by spreading them on a cookie sheet and putting them in the oven at 400°F for two hours. This gives the roots a rich, warm, almost chocolaty flavor that makes a pretty good coffee substitute, especially when topped with a little cinnamon.

DANDELION VINEGAR

Makes 3 ½ cups
*Prep time: 10 minutes, plus 4 to 6
weeks to steep*

Apple cider vinegar is becoming more
and more popular, with a long list
of health benefits on its own before
we even add the herbs! Vinegar is
an easy way to add the vitamins and
minerals packed into all parts of this
plant into all kinds of dishes. You
can also just take a tablespoon of the
vinegar mixed in a little water. Use
this with oil to dress a salad, spritz on
cooked veggies, or deglaze a pan and
make a light sauce for meat.

INGREDIENTS

1 cup fresh dandelion roots, washed
　and coarsely chopped
1 cup dandelion leaves, torn into
　small pieces
1 cup dandelion flowers
1 quart apple cider vinegar

SUPPLIES

a large jar

1. Put all the botanicals into a jar.

2. Cover with the apple cider
vinegar.

3. Line the lid with plastic wrap or
wax paper (vinegar will corrode a
metal top) and let steep in a cool,
dry place for 4 to 6 weeks.

4. When steeping is done, strain
the vinegar and use in any dish
you desire.

DANDELION CHAI BLEND

Makes 40 cups
Prep time: 1 hour 25 minutes
(30 minutes active)

All of the spices in the delicious chai are immune stimulating and antibiotic, and many are antiviral and anti-inflammatory. Mixed together, they make for a spicy, sweet, comforting treat.

INGREDIENTS

1 cup dandelion root, cut into uniform
   small pieces

2 tablespoons whole peppercorns

3 tablespoons cardamom pods

3 tablespoons cinnamon chips

¼ cup dried ginger pieces

1 cup black tea leaves (use rooibos if you
   prefer decaf)

½ cup dried dandelion leaves, crumbled

2 vanilla beans, cut into small pieces

Honey and light cream or half-and-half,
   for serving

SUPPLIES

a baking sheet

a food processor or coffee grinder

an airtight container

a muslin bag or tea ball

1. Arrange the dandelion root pieces in a single layer on a baking sheet. Roast in a 200°F oven for 30 minutes, or until they turn dark brown and are completely dried.

2. In a mini food processor or coffee grinder, process the peppercorns, cardamom pods, cinnamon chips, and ginger pieces until you have uniform small bits. Mix in the black tea, dandelion leaves, and vanilla beans until well combined. Store the tea blend in an airtight container until ready to use.

3. For each cup of tea you want to make, use 1 teaspoon of the tea blend. Bring water to a boil in a saucepan and add the tea blend in a tea ball or muslin bag. Cover and let steep for 15 to 20 minutes. Remove the tea blend and serve the tea in mugs with honey and light cream or half-and-half.

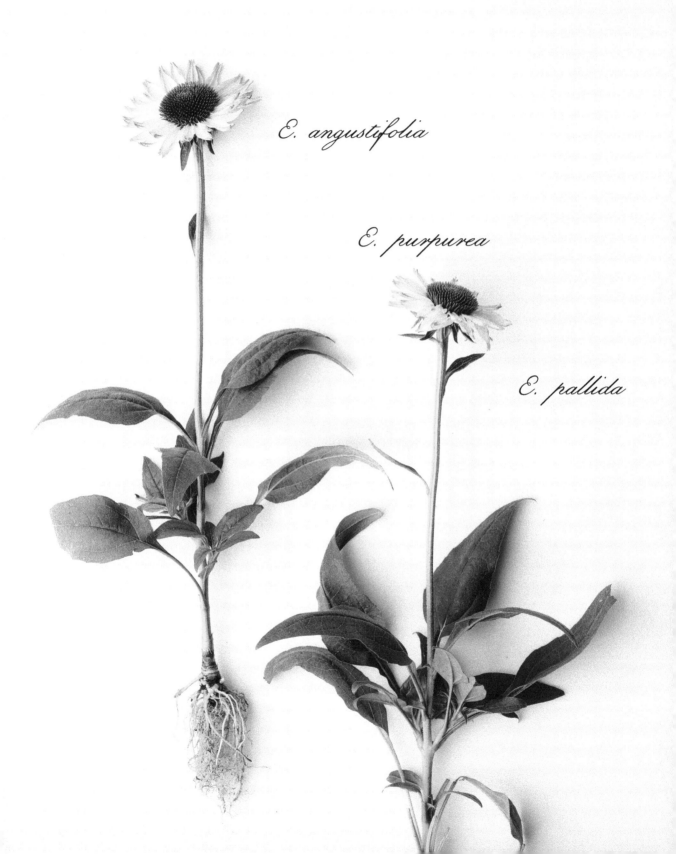

E. angustifolia

E. purpurea

E. pallida

ECHINACEA

Echinacea just might have been the single herb that led to the current renaissance in herbal medicine. In the late 1980s and early 1990s, word of this plant spread like wildfire, like a secret password to a special club. I still remember the first time I heard about it at our quaint little shop filled with teas, potpourris, and sweet pillows. A customer asked for it, and as was our custom back in those days, we listened, nodded, and, upon arriving home, tore into our books to learn more about this presumably magical herb that could prevent the common cold. Interestingly, the name is derived from the Greek word *echinos*, which means "sea urchin," referring to echinacea's sea urchin-like, cone-shaped seed head.

ABOUT ECHINACEA

OTHER COMMON NAMES purple cone-flower, snakeroot, black sampson, red sunflower, Indian head

SAFETY CONSIDERATIONS may cause upset stomach or diarrhea when used in large doses

PARTS USED roots and all aerial parts

ENERGETICS bitter, cool, dry

PROPERTIES Echinacea is antibacterial, anti-catarrhal, antifungal, anti-inflammatory, antioxidant, antiseptic, antitumor, antiviral, astringent, carminative, fever-reducing, and pain-relieving. It moves the body toward health, stimulates and supports the immune system, promotes secretion of saliva and perspiration, and is a digestive, purifier, stimulant, and wound healer.

USES Echinacea can help heal tooth-aches, snakebites, stings, allergies, wounds, burns, joint pain, sore throats, coughs, colds, and infections. It boosts the immune system and attacks general infection; treats weeping wounds, boils, abscesses, urinary tract infections, and enlarged lymph glands; promotes skin regeneration; and ameliorates psoriasis. You can take it both internally and externally for many of these afflictions, thereby multiplying the effects. In my experience, to ward off illness, you must take echinacea at the very first sign of a viral assault, be it a scratchy throat or an achy arm muscle (my own tip-off). Take it early, often, and in a form that will be effective, like a capsule or tincture.

PREPARATIONS Echinacea is available as tinctures, capsules, cough drops, syrups, and teas from the root, leaves, and/or flowers. Salves, poultices, and compresses are effective forms for external use. If you are able to grow it, do. Having fresh echinacea at the ready comes in very handy.

DOSAGE When used internally, it is best to pulse, meaning to use it for about 10 days and then stop for a few days to let the immune system rest before resuming usage. Ingest as tolerated when illness threatens. Take large doses for acute infection.

PREPARATION TIP Every year I pull a plant and clean the roots carefully before grinding them, along with some leaves and a flower or two, to mix with high-proof vodka in a jar. A good tincture made with fresh roots will have a little tingle on the tongue.

Home treatments

Echinacea is a very good treatment for nasty spider bites. Prepare a poultice of 1 teaspoon echinacea tincture and 1 teaspoon of a drawing clay, such as bentonite or green clay. Add just enough water, if necessary, to create a paste. Use this paste on the bite two or three times a day and alternate with 15-minute soaks in water with Epsom salts. Some spider venom can destroy tissue in the area of the bite, so if there isn't significant improvement within a few days, see a physician. Most of the time, these bites can be treated at home.

For upper-respiratory illness, the cool, dry energetics of echinacea work well to help a hot, sweaty, mucus-laden situation. Echinacea blends well with the energetics of thyme and sage to dry and warm up the system. A vinegar or honey made with those three herbs is good to have on hand for your next cough or cold.

ECHINACEA-ELDERBERRY GUMMIES

Makes 64 (1-inch) pieces
Prep time: 45 minutes

Kids love these. It can be tough to get everyone on board the immunity train, especially if they think something is medicine—a spoonful of sugar can make all the difference. These herbs will go a long way toward keeping viruses at bay.

INGREDIENTS

2 cups elderberry juice (see Tip)

¼ cup freshly squeezed lemon juice

1 cup echinacea roots, leaves, and
   flowers, chopped

4 tablespoons unflavored powdered gelatin

5 tablespoons sugar

SUPPLIES

2 saucepans

a square glass baking dish

an airtight container

TIP To make elderberry juice, combine 2 cups of ripe fresh elderberries with ½ cup of water in a saucepan. Simmer over medium heat, until the berries burst and release their heat. Mash the berries, then strain through a fine-mesh strainer or muslin bag. Add more water if necessary to get 2 cups of liquid.

1. In a medium saucepan, combine the elderberry juice, lemon juice, and echinacea, and simmer over low heat until the liquid is reduced by about half. Set aside to cool. Strain out the echinacea.

2. In another saucepan, combine the well-cooled liquid with the gelatin and sugar. Cook over low heat, stirring often, until the gelatin and sugar dissolve completely, about 3 minutes.

3. Skim any foam from the surface.

4. Pour the mixture into a lightly oiled square glass baking dish, to be cut into 1-inch squares. If you have silicone candy molds, even better. Refrigerate until the mixture sets, about 10 minutes. Store in an airtight container at room temperature for 5 days or in the refrigerator for 2 weeks.

IMMUNITEA

Makes 50 (1-cup) servings
Prep time: 30 minutes

Drink this tea one to three times per day when you feel the very beginnings of illness coming on, or when you're heading into an immuno-compromised situation, such as traveling by plane or otherwise sharing space with sick people. Continue drinking for up to 2 weeks if needed.

INGREDIENTS

1 cup echinacea

1 cup elderberry

½ cup rosehips

½ cup astragalus

2 teaspoons grated fresh ginger

Honey and lemon, for serving

SUPPLIES

a food processor or coffee grinder

a jar or airtight container

a tea ball or muslin bag

1. In a mini food processor or coffee grinder, grind all the ingredients to small, similarly sized pieces. Mix together well and store the tea blend in a jar or other airtight container until ready to use.

2. For each cup of tea you want to make, use 1 tablespoon of the tea blend. Bring water to a boil in a saucepan, add the tea blend in a tea ball or muslin bag (or simmer loose and strain through a wire-mesh strainer just prior to drinking), then simmer on low heat for ½ hour or more.

3. Pour into mugs and add honey and lemon as desired.

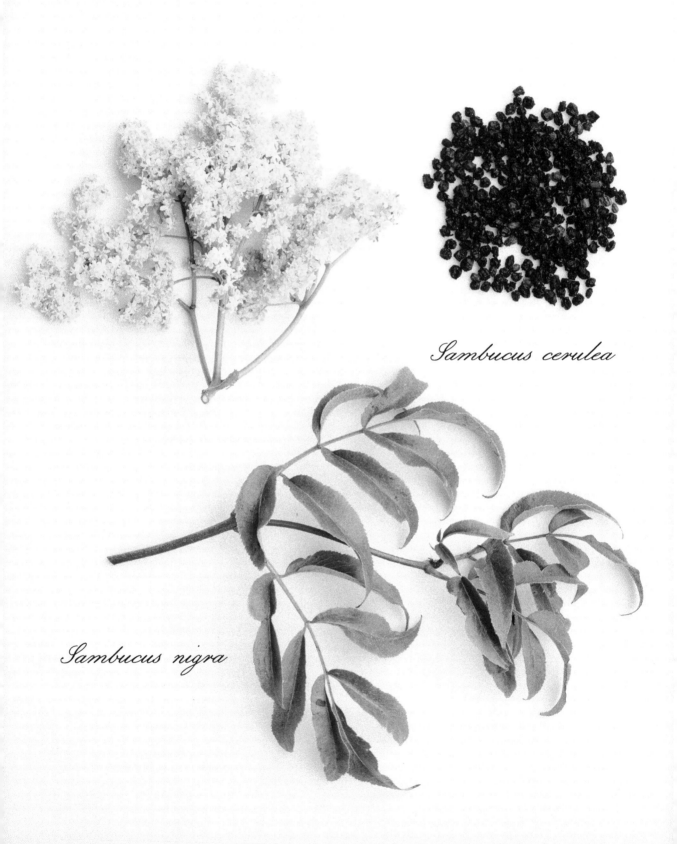

Sambucus cerulea

Sambucus nigra

ELDER

I've grown elder in my yard for 25 years. I wouldn't enter winter without it! The elder keeps us healthy, and there are several varieties. In the eastern United States, we have the dark, purplish-black elderberries. The western states have powdery-blue berries and a red variety (*Sambucus racemosa*) that some say are fine to use after cooking and others say are poisonous. I'd avoid them and use the blue elderberries that are known to be safe. The elder recipes in this section are medicinal, but you can sneak elderberry into pie, jelly, wine, and candy.

ABOUT ELDER

OTHER COMMON NAMES Elderberry, black elder, European elder, European elderberry, European black elderberry, blue elderberry, and Mexican elderberry. Tapiro flowers are sometimes referred to as elder blow.

SAFETY CONSIDERATIONS Only the ripe berries and flowers are edible. The leaves, stems and unripe berries contain cyanide-inducing glycosides, which can cause a toxic buildup of cyanide in the body. Large quantities of uncooked berries may cause illness due to the glycosides in the tiny seeds. Heating the berries renders them harmless.

PARTS USED berries and flowers for internal use; leaves and flowers for external use

ENERGETICS The flowers and berries are bitter, drying, cool, slightly sweet.

PROPERTIES Some herbalists prefer the flowers to the berries due to their antiseptic, antispasmodic, antiviral, diaphoretic, diuretic, and styptic properties. The berries are antiviral, diaphoretic, diuretic, and laxative. Elderberries are also a good source of anthocyanins, which are powerful antioxidants. The berries contain vitamins A and C, calcium, thiamine, niacin, potassium, and protein. They are thought to make cells slippery so that viruses cannot attach and replicate, warding off and shortening the duration of viral infections. The leaves are emollient, pain-relieving, and vulnerary.

USES Elderflower tea is a time-tested remedy for upper-respiratory infections. It loosens and moves stuck mucus in cases of bronchitis or sinusitis. Berries and flowers ward off colds and flu. Elder's diuretic and anti-inflammatory properties explain its use for rheumatic and arthritic conditions. Elder leaf, used topically, is known to help soothe and heal wounds, cuts, burns, and swollen bruises.

PREPARATIONS You can make or find tinctures, teas, syrups, flower essences, and wine. You can use the berries in all types of jelly, baked goods, wine, cough drops, and candy. The leaves are often used in salves.

DOSAGE A slice or two of pie contains at least a cup of the berries, meaning the berries are very safe. With the flowers, it's safe to drink the tea or use the tincture several times a day.

HARVESTING TIP When the berries ripen, it can be overwhelming to harvest them all. Some go directly into the freezer in the right quantity for syrup, while the bulk are made into juice by heating them with a little lemon juice.

Home treatments

Elderberry is best known for its effectiveness against the flu. Several studies (most often specifically using elderberry extracts in Sambucol® products) show flu patients recovering in two to three days if they start using the products early and often. I haven't had the flu since learning of elder. One year my mother and uncle were not so lucky and got hit hard. I insisted that they begin using elderberry. Before it was time for the second dose after just four hours, they both felt human again. They were much better by the next day. Trust me, it works!

Elder works in a similar way for colds or any sort of viral infection.

ELDERBERRY LIQUEUR

Makes about 6 cups
Prep time: 1 hour 10 minutes
(10 minutes active), plus at least 1
month to age

With elderberry, medicine doesn't
have to taste bad. A small glass of this
liqueur sipped each evening during
winter will go a long way toward
keeping you healthy and happy, and
is a delicious way to unwind after a
long day.

INGREDIENTS

1 quart fresh elderberries

2 cups sugar

Zest and juice of 1 lemon

1 (750 mL) bottle 80-proof vodka

SUPPLIES

a 2-quart container

some glass bottles

1. In a bowl, using a potato masher or pestle, crush the elderberries and sugar together. Let stand for about 1 hour.

2. Add the lemon zest and lemon juice.

3. Transfer the mixture to a clean 2-quart container and add the vodka.

4. Cover and let age in a cool, dark place for 1 month.

5. After a month, use a fine-mesh strainer to strain out the solids; discard the solids.

6. Transfer the liqueur to pretty glass bottles.

7. You can enjoy this liqueur immediately, but the flavor does continue to develop over time. For the best flavor, age the liqueur for at least another month.

ELDER SYRUP

Makes about 2 quarts
Prep time: 1 hour

In this version of elderberry syrup, the brandy is mostly used as a slight preservative. You can omit it or double it as preferred. This syrup is tasty enough that kids ask for it, and it can be used as a tea sweetener, on pancakes, on ice cream, etc. It can also be used as a condiment for food, making it a very convenient way to add elder to the family diet. During an illness, take 1 tablespoon of the syrup four times a day.

INGREDIENTS

2 quarts elderberries

2½ pounds sugar

1 cup dried elderflowers

1½ teaspoons ground cloves

1 tablespoon small cinnamon chips

1 cup brandy

SUPPLIES

saucepans

a mesh strainer or cheesecloth

some bottles or jars

1. In a saucepan over medium heat, cook the elderberries for a few minutes, until they start to burst.

2. Mash the berries with the back of a large spoon to release their juices.

3. Using a mesh strainer or several layers of cheesecloth (or a square of old clean T-shirt), strain the juice. You'll need about 1 quart.

4. In a large saucepan, combine the juice with the sugar, elder-flowers, cloves, and cinnamon chips. Simmer over low heat for 20 minutes.

5. Remove from the heat, let cool, then strain to remove the solids.

6. Once the syrup has cooled, add the brandy. Pour the finished syrup into bottles or jars and store in the refrigerator for a year.

TIP You can put spices and flowers into a sachet or muslin bag to avoid straining a second time.

Allium sativum

GARLIC

In *A Midsummer Night's Dream*, Bottom instructs, "And most, dear actors, eat no onions or garlic, for we are to utter sweet breath."

Some people are convinced that garlic works primarily by keeping other people far away. There's something to be said for that, as garlic is pungent and lingers on the breath, sometimes veritably seeping from the pores, but there's more to the healing powers of garlic. It produces a chemical called allicin (one of 30 some sulfur compounds) that's released when garlic is crushed, chopped, or chewed. This releases several other sulfur compounds that all work together to heal and promote health. If only everyone ate it every day, then nobody would be annoyed by the scent!

ABOUT GARLIC

OTHER COMMON NAMES stinking rose, Italian perfume, Russian penicillin, poor man's treacle, Bronx vanilla.

SAFETY CONSIDERATIONS If you're on blood-thinning medication, check with your doctor before taking garlic medicinally. Also let your physician know about garlic supplementation prior to surgery so they can tell you when to stop taking it. Garlic supplementation (above dietary use) should be avoided during pregnancy. Garlic may cause contact dermatitis with overuse.

PARTS USED bulbs, cloves, scapes, flowers

ENERGETICS all (what does that tell you?)

PROPERTIES Garlic is antibacterial, antibiotic, antifungal, anti-inflammatory, antiviral, vulnerary, and immune-boosting. It clears arteries, thins blood, heals wounds, treats lung ailments, and combats bacteria and yeast.

USES The uses for garlic are nearly limitless; entire books have been written on the subject. It is touted for everything from colds to cancer, and currently shows great promise for MRSA infections. It helps fight coughs, heart ailments, high blood pressure, and high cholesterol, and regulates blood sugar. Anecdotally, people have used it warmed as "sweet oil" (olive oil infused with garlic) for earaches. Garlic can also be used on external infections. Diallyl sulfide and diallyl trisulfide are two of hundreds of compounds in garlic that are being studied for circulatory improvement, cardiac health, and applications for cancer patients. Eating garlic can also prevent flea, tick, and mosquito bites.

PREPARATIONS Garlic can be used in juice, capsules, pills, tinctures, infused oils, and fresh in food. Here in Pennsylvania Dutch country, you can also find garlic jelly! Fresh raw garlic is the best.

DOSAGE Follow the directions on commercial products. During illness, it's safe to take three or more cloves daily. The upper limit is about 10 cloves or the equivalent.

GROWING TIP Garlic is easy to grow and doesn't take much space. If you have a source of organic garlic, purchase a bulb to grow. Plant in autumn or early spring, in a sunny location with well-drained soil. Plant root-side down 4 to 6 inches apart in rows 1½ to 2 inches apart. Cover with 2 inches of dirt. Mulch for winter.

Home treatments

For stubborn colds, garlic honey comes in handy. My sister makes it by chopping and dumping three or four whole bulbs and a lemon into a jar of honey. It sounds terrible, and I only like it when I'm sick. It's good in tea or right out of the jar, and works fast.

If you have a teen in the house, the same honey, with the garlic crushed fine into a paste, helps with pimples and acne. Apply about a tablespoon to a clean face and leave on the skin for 10 or 15 minutes. Doing this regularly will clear and brighten the skin.

BASIL PESTO WITH FRESH GARLIC

Makes 2 cups
Prep time: 10 minutes

The first time I had this pesto was on the deck at a friend's A-frame house in the Adirondacks. She threw it together after a long day of hiking and exploring, and served it with steamed shrimp over linguine. I've been hooked ever since.

INGREDIENTS

4 cups fresh basil leaves

6 cloves garlic

¾ cup toasted pine nuts

1 cup olive oil

¾ cup Parmesan cheese, freshly grated

SUPPLIES

a food processor

an airtight container

1. Place the basil leaves, garlic, and pine nuts in a food processor. Slowly add the olive oil and process to a chunky paste. Add more oil if needed. Fold in the cheese.

2. Store the pesto in an airtight container for up to 1 week in the refrigerator or for up to 6 months in the freezer.

TIP You can use other herbs, such as chickweed, dandelion leaves, catnip, nettles, parsley, or sage, in place of or in addition to the basil. And try different nuts or seeds, like walnuts, sunflower seeds, pumpkin seeds, macadamia nuts, cashews, or pecans, to mix up the flavor.

GARLIC AND HERB OXYMEL

Makes 1 quart
Prep time: 30 minutes, plus at least 1 week to steep

The term *oxymel* is from the Latin *oxymeli*, meaning acid and honey. This is a splendid medium that lends itself well to many different herbal uses. Vinegars extract vitamins and minerals as well as the other various herbal properties. The vinegar itself is the preservative, and oxymels can be used alone as medicine, diluted with hot tea or water to ward off or recover from illness, or incorporated into dressings or marinades for meals.

INGREDIENTS

2½ cups apple cider vinegar

1 cup honey

1 head garlic, cloves peeled and minced

1 tablespoon fresh thyme leaves

1 tablespoon chopped fresh rosemary

1 tablespoon grated fresh ginger

SUPPLIES

a 1-quart jar

1. In a 1-quart jar, stir together the apple cider vinegar and honey until the honey is mostly dissolved.

2. Add the garlic, thyme, rosemary, and ginger.

3. Cover the jar with a nonmetallic cap or lay plastic wrap across the top and then secure the lid. Let steep at room temperature for at least 1 week, shaking the jar daily, before using.

TIP I like to leave the herbs and spices in the oxymel, but you can also strain them out if you prefer.

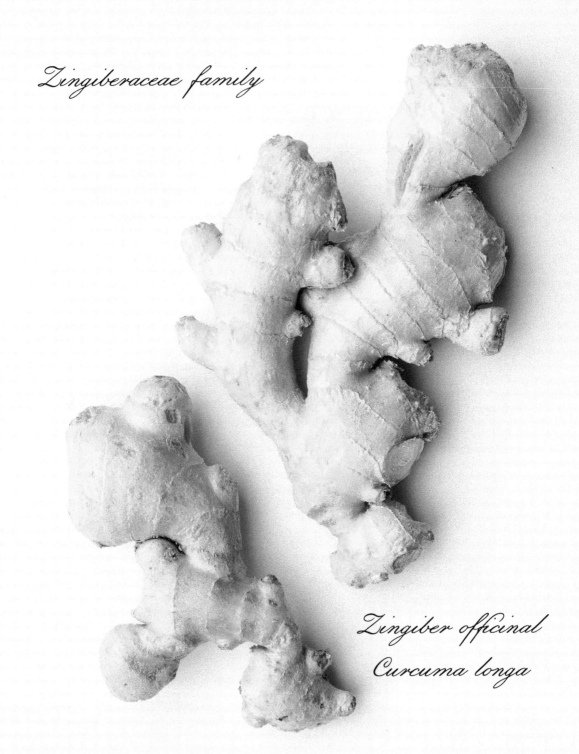

Zingiberaceae family

Zingiber officinal

Curcuma longa

GINGER

Popular for both baking and cooking, ginger has been in use for more than 5,000 years. It was initially cultivated in China before spreading throughout Southeast Asia, India, West Africa, and the Caribbean Islands. Ginger ale is a traditional home remedy for an upset stomach, and ginger tea is gaining popularity for the same reason. There are many varieties of ginger, including turmeric and galangal. They all have similar properties, yet each has unique healing benefits as well.

ABOUT GINGER

OTHER COMMON NAME gingerroot

SAFETY CONSIDERATIONS Avoid regular supplementation if taking anticoagulant medication.

PART USED root

ENERGETICS pungent, hot, and sweet

PROPERTIES Ginger is anti-inflammatory, antibacterial, antifungal, antiviral, carminative, diaphoretic, immune-boosting, thermogenic, and blood-thinning. It is currently being studied for its ability to lower blood glucose levels, increase insulin sensitivity, lower cholesterol, and help with other serious conditions.

USES Ginger is best known for its ability to help nausea, including sea sickness, chemotherapy-related nausea, nausea after surgery, and morning sickness in pregnancy. It also stimulates digestion, causing the stomach to empty faster while soothing and relaxing the entire system. Ginger may also help with menstrual pain, migraine headaches, and gum health. Regular use of ginger may help relieve pain and swelling from osteoarthritis, rheumatoid arthritis, and muscular pains. Turmeric is currently the darling of the superfood set; it shows a lot of promise for many diseases and is specifically good for joint pain.

PREPARATIONS Ginger is available fresh, dried, powdered, juiced, candied, and as tinctures, teas, syrups, and essential oils.

DOSAGE In cooking, ginger is considered to be quite safe when used in moderation. Tinctures, teas, and syrups may be used three to four times a day. It's important to properly dilute ginger essential oils.

GROWING TIP You can grow ginger indoors as long as you have a very warm spot, like a window with clear southern exposure. Give each plant a 12- to 18-inch pot with good drainage. Place trimmed rhizomes eye- or bud-up, and cover with an inch or so of good dirt.

Home treatments

I wish I had known about ginger when I was pregnant with my daughter—crystallized ginger can be a lifesaver for morning sickness (although it doesn't work for everyone, sadly). Now I often give expecting mothers a bag of crystallized ginger to get them through early pregnancy.

I recently had a cousin going on a cruise through Alaskan waters who was worried about seasickness. We gave her a jar of ginger capsules. She was doubtful, but one day on the ship she got so desperate she tried them. Shortly afterward, she was the only one on deck who wasn't some shade of sickly green.

All the terrific protective properties of ginger also work topically. Ginger kills bacteria that cause acne and blemishes and brings blood circulation to the skin, improving tone and getting rid of dead cells. Combine finely grated ginger, olive oil, and sugar in about equal parts; scoop a bit onto your fingers and scrub wherever you'd like smoother, fresher skin, avoiding the eye area. Rinse and shower as normal. I particularly love this in winter because it revives dry skin.

TRIPLE GINGER ELIXIR

Makes about 3 cups
Prep time: 30 minutes, plus about 1
month to steep

This is a delicious drink to sip after dinner and also packs a powerful medicinal punch—you can take it by the tablespoonful when you're sick. Added to some hot tea, you can reap all the incredible benefits of ginger by the mugful. The ingredients are very flexible, so if you can't find one or two of them, don't let that stop you. As long as you have ginger, honey, and lemon, you're good to go.

INGREDIENTS

½ cup chopped fresh ginger

¼ cup chopped fresh turmeric

1½ tablespoons dried galangal pieces
   (¼ cup fresh, if you can find it)

1 lemon, thinly sliced

1 tablespoon cinnamon stick pieces

2 star anise

5 cardamom pods

1 cup honey

2 to 3 cups 100-proof vodka or brandy

SUPPLIES

a 1-quart jar

1. In a 1-quart jar, combine the ginger, turmeric, galangal, lemon slices, cinnamon, star anise, cardamom pods, and honey. Pour in enough of the vodka to completely cover the ingredients.

2. Cover the jar and let steep for about a month.

3. Strain and enjoy. Store in a cool place out of direct sunlight.

GOLDEN MILK TEA

Makes about 12 ounces
Prep time: 20 minutes

Golden milk is a delicious treat to drink in the evening and imparts all of the glorious health benefits of turmeric and ginger. Turmeric in particular is activated when mixed with black pepper and fats, which shows how this traditional Ayurvedic recipe has survived the test of time.

INGREDIENTS

2 cups water

¼ pound fresh turmeric roots, grated (wear gloves for this)

1 (1-inch) piece fresh ginger, grated

1 tablespoon ground cinnamon

2 teaspoons freshly ground black pepper

½ teaspoon ground nutmeg

3 teaspoons coconut oil

1 cup milk of your choice (dairy, soy, or nut)

1 heaping teaspoon honey

SUPPLIES

rubber gloves

saucepans

an airtight jar

1. In a saucepan over high heat, bring the water to a boil, then reduce the heat to low and simmer for 5 minutes.

2. Add the turmeric, ginger, cinnamon, pepper, nutmeg, and coconut oil, and stir while simmering for a few more minutes, or until the liquid forms a paste.

3. In another saucepan, warm the milk over low heat.

4. Add a heaping teaspoon of the paste and the honey. Stir to mix well before drinking.

5. The leftover paste will keep in an airtight jar in the refrigerator for up to 2 weeks.

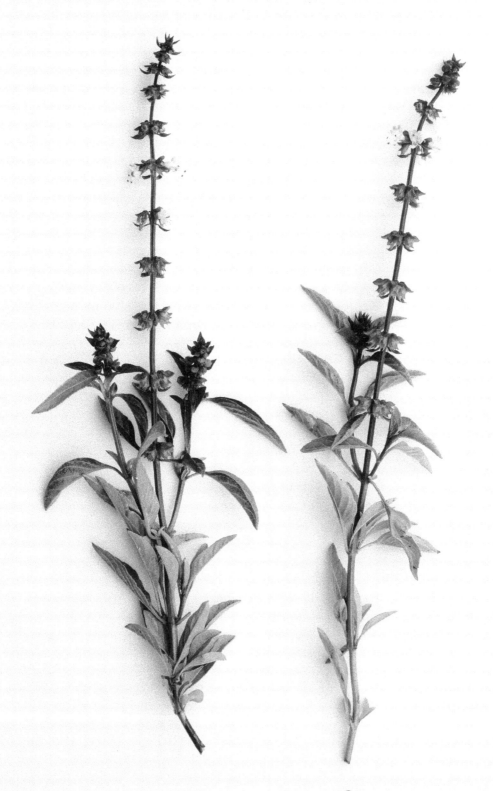

Ocimum tenuiflorum

HOLY BASIL

Holy basil, or tulsi, has long been revered in the Hindu religion. Many Indian families keep a holy basil plant in the courtyard next to the house, worshipping it morning and night. Holy basil falls under the grouping of herbs used in Rasayana, the Ayurvedic path to optimal, glowing health, rejuvenation, and longevity. Who doesn't want that?

For thousands of years, holy basil has been considered one of the top healing plants in India, and fortunately it made its way West in the past few decades. Its versatility has made it a recent favorite of mine.

ABOUT HOLY BASIL

OTHER COMMON NAMES tulsi, tulasi, *Ocimum sanctum*, Indian basil, the incomparable one, hot basil, queen of herbs, sacred basil

SAFETY CONSIDERATIONS If you're taking an anticoagulant, check with your physician before using holy basil. Stop use of the herb prior to surgery. Hypoglycemic people may experience drops in blood sugar and should use caution with holy basil.

PARTS USED all aerial parts

ENERGETICS hot and cooling, pungent and sweet

PROPERTIES In some cultures, holy basil is believed to have, on a spiritual level, the ability to balance chakras, clear negative energies, and promote an open heart. It is adaptogenic, analgesic, antibacterial, antifungal, anti-inflammatory, antioxidant, antiviral, carminative, antidepressive, diuretic, expectorant, grounding, nervine, neuroprotective, and tonic. It reduces fever and supports the immune system.

USES Holy basil is used for anxiety, asthma, colds, bronchitis, depression, diabetes, earache, eczema, flu, headache, hives, stomach upset, heart disease, fever, ringworm, and stress. It is also used as a mosquito repellent.

PREPARATIONS Teas, tinctures, fresh leaves, and capsules. Externally, you can use essential oil and hydrosol. Note that oils must either be strongly diluted or diffused.

DOSAGE Holy basil is considered a very safe herb, and can be ingested up to four times a day. Some women feel it is too hot and prefer to blend it with other herbs, such as rose.

GROWING TIP In my region, zone 6b, holy basil grows as an annual. In tropical climates it will grow like shrubs with woody stems. I usually plant a short row of holy basil plants, but be warned—birds love them. I cover mine with netting until they are about 8 to 10 inches tall; otherwise the birds will get to them before I do!

Home treatments

My personal experience with holy basil has been profound. A friend, Sandi Wakefield from Black Kat Herbs, recommended it to me at a time when I was floundering and drowning under some massive responsibility and anxiety. I had grown and tinctured holy basil that summer, so I tried it. I took a single dose, and 15 minutes later I was able to look at everything objectively and could start working to resolve things with more clarity.

Holy basil is a powerful antiviral and supports the immune system, making it a good choice to take daily as a preventive. When the body is managing stress effectively, it is easier to fight off viral, bacterial, or fungal infections. Everything just works better with holy basil.

TONIC GRANOLA BARS WITH HOLY BASIL, ASTRAGALUS, AND ASHWAGANDHA

Makes 8 to 10 bars
Prep time: 90 minutes
(30 minutes active)

These granola bars are great to grab for breakfast when you're on the run— they're delicious and provide a terrific boost. No baking required!

INGREDIENTS

4 tablespoons (½ stick) butter, plus more for greasing

2 cups quick oats

1 cup crispy rice cereal

¼ cup peanuts

¼ cup pumpkin seeds or pistachios

¼ cup mini chocolate chips

1 tablespoon holy basil powder

1 tablespoon astragalus root powder

1 tablespoon ashwagandha root powder

1 tablespoon minced crystallized ginger

¼ teaspoon salt

¼ cup brown sugar

¼ cup honey

½ cup peanut butter

1 teaspoon vanilla extract

SUPPLIES

a baking pan

a large saucepan

an airtight container

1. Butter a 9-inch square baking pan.

2. In a large bowl, stir together the oats, cereal, peanuts, pumpkin seeds, chocolate chips, herb powders, ginger, and salt. Set aside.

3. In a large saucepan, bring the butter, brown sugar, honey, and peanut butter to a low boil for a few minutes. Remove from the heat and stir in the vanilla extract, followed by the dry ingredients. Mix completely.

4. Spread the mixture evenly in the prepared baking pan and refrigerate for an hour before cutting and serving.

5. The granola bars can be stored in an airtight container in the refrigerator for up to 10 days.

TULSI ROSE TEA BLEND

Makes about 30 cups
Prep time: 15 minutes

This is a bright, flavorful herbal tea that tastes good and is both cheering and antiviral. I really like to trim, zest, and dry the lemon peel myself, although you can buy this commercially. Everything else comes from the summer garden or the farmers' market.

INGREDIENTS

½ cup holy basil

¼ cup rose petals

2 tablespoons spearmint leaves

2 tablespoons elderberries

1 tablespoon dried lemon zest

SUPPLIES

a jar and a tea ball

1. In a jar, blend together all the ingredients. The elderberries tend to sink to the bottom, so keep that in mind when filling a tea ball.

2. For each cup of tea, put a heaping teaspoon of the blend in a tea ball, place it in a mug, and pour hot water into the mug. Steep for 5 to 10 minutes. You can remove the herbs or let them continue to steep while you drink.

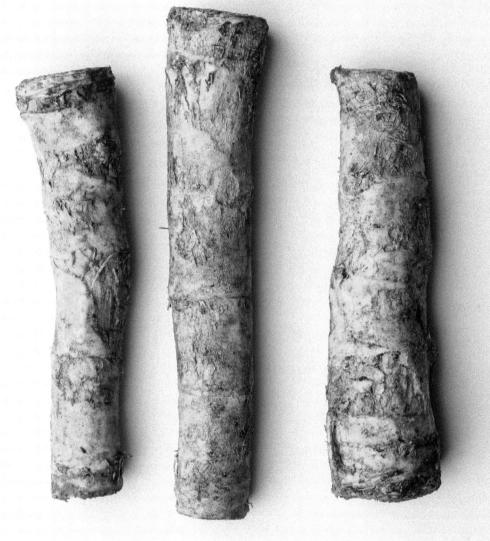

Armoracia rusticana

HORSERADISH

I don't know why horseradish isn't more popular. It's delicious on meats, vegetables, potatoes, and seafood, yet is rarely used as an everyday food. Hot sauces and spicy dishes have really gained a foothold in the U.S., but somehow this health-giving root has been largely left out of these products. When horseradish is cut, cells are crushed, causing enzymes and glucosides to interact, releasing the oil, which explains why horseradish root has no smell until it is cut, grated, or ground. Grinding horseradish is a memorable, sinus-opening experience that might be best done outside. If you don't have this centuries-old remedy growing in your garden, consider adding it; otherwise, the roots can easily be found at your local supermarket.

ABOUT HORSERADISH

OTHER COMMON NAME stingnose

SAFETY CONSIDERATIONS Horseradish essential oil is classified as a hazardous substance, and the juice can cause blistering, so check skin frequently when using the root in a poultice.

PARTS USED fresh root, small young leaves, and flowers

ENERGETICS spicy and hot

PROPERTIES Horseradish contains a surprising number of helpful properties, including being antibiotic, anti-inflammatory, antimicrobial, antioxidant, antiviral, diaphoretic, diuretic, expectorant, and stimulating. It contains important nutrients, including vitamin C, calcium, iron, magnesium, phosphorus, potassium, and zinc.

USES Horseradish stimulates the gallbladder's release of bile, making it a great alternative for digestive problems. The heat of the horseradish is different from capsicum (see page 55), and we feel it most sharply in our sinuses, rather than in our mouths. This gets all the mucus running and helps loosen and expel sinus congestion. All head colds and stuck upper-respiratory infections respond to horseradish. It is also helpful with arthritis, urinary tract infections, headaches, kidney stones, fluid retention, cough, bronchitis, sore muscles, sciatic nerve pain, and gout. Horseradish is thought to detoxify the liver. Syrups help hoarseness or bronchitis specifically but are useful for other applications as well.

Young leaves can be used as instant poultices for headaches and laid directly on the forehead. The fresh flowers may be made into a tea as an antiviral and a mild decongestant.

PREPARATIONS You can make syrups, tinctures, and vinegars. The only things available commercially seem to be fresh sauces or processed grated fresh horseradish root, which are widely available in grocery stores.

DOSAGE Horseradish is safe to use as tolerated. The equivalent of ½ teaspoon grated horseradish makes an adult dose.

GROWING TIP Horseradish is easy to grow, and it will spread. In some cases it can be downright invasive. Mine is in the shade, and while it has increased from one crown to about six over a decade, that's not terrible. Never rototill horseradish.

Home treatments

For joint pain, a horseradish poultice opens capillaries and brings blood to the area, increasing circulation and reddening the skin. Make the compress by grating enough fresh horseradish to cover the intended area with a layer about ¼ inch thick. Mix with enough water to make a thick paste. Apply the paste to a piece of cloth (flannel works well) at least twice as large as the area. Place the cloth on the area. Once it begins to burn, remove the cloth. Check the skin every few minutes to be sure it isn't blistering.

Horseradish is considered one of the strongest herbal diuretics, and with its antibiotic properties, it is a terrific choice for kidney disease, bladder issues, or urinary tract infections. Half a teaspoon of freshly grated horseradish three times a day will help flush out these infections.

HORSERADISH VODKA

Makes 1 quart
Prep time: 45 minutes

You can use this as the alcohol in a Bloody Mary or mix it with just a swallow of juice to get its healing benefits. This recipe is a good way to preserve horseradish instead of making a ton of cocktail sauce or jars of horseradish mixed in vinegar.

INGREDIENTS

1 (8-inch) piece fresh horseradish root, finely grated

24 ounces 100-proof vodka

SUPPLIES

a 1-quart bottle

1. Let the grated horseradish rest for about 10 minutes to allow the oils to release and the "heat" to develop.

2. Place the horseradish into a 1-quart bottle. Fill with the vodka (no need to strain). Store in a cool, dry place.

3. Before using, give the bottle a good shake. Use the horseradish vodka in a mixed drink or as a dose of medicine.

FIRE CIDER

Makes about 1 quart
Prep time: 45 minutes, plus at least 2 weeks to steep

This cider is based on Rosemary Gladstar's recipe, with a few personal additions. The amounts listed aren't critical, and you can add or delete anything you want. Many people take a shot of this every day, particularly when there are a lot of bugs going around. Another way to use it is by mixing it with water or juice. It can also be blended with a little oil for a salad dressing.

INGREDIENTS

1 quart apple cider vinegar (see Tip)

5 hot peppers, chopped

1 large red onion, chopped

⅓ cup dried or 1 cup fresh elderberries

3 slices astragalus, chopped

½ cup grated fresh horseradish

1 head garlic, peeled and chopped

¼ cup grated fresh ginger

1 tablespoon ground or 3 tablespoons grated fresh turmeric

Juice of 1 lemon

1 cup honey

Water or juice, for serving

SUPPLIES

a half-gallon container

1. Place the apple cider vinegar, peppers, onion, elderberries, astragalus, horseradish, garlic, ginger, turmeric, and lemon juice in a half gallon container and secure with a nonmetallic lid.

2. Let steep in a warm, dry place for at least 2 weeks.

3. Strain, then add the honey to the vinegar.

4. To use, dilute the cider with water or juice, and down the hatch!

TIP Be sure that the vinegar is true apple cider vinegar with the "mother"—the healthy bacteria that gives it a cloudy appearance.

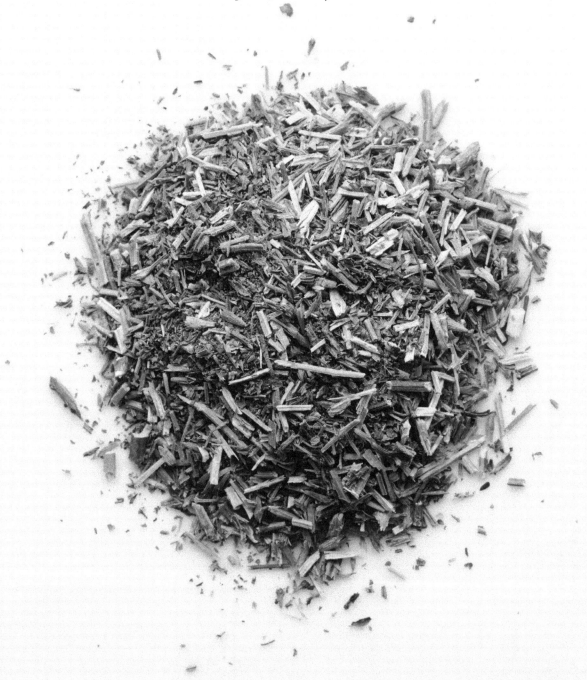

Hyssopus officinalis

HYSSOP

Hyssop has been used for centuries, probably millennia. European settlers brought the plant to the U.S. It has medicinal properties, many culinary uses, and brewing uses (such as in absinthe and chartreuse), and is valued for its fragrance, used as a scent in soaps and other products. It's also beautiful fresh and makes a gorgeous addition to a flower arrangement. In some places, hyssop is a ditch weed, growing with wild abandon along roadsides and in meadows. I have yet to find it in my area, but it is hardy in USDA growing zones 4 through 10. It is a shrubby perennial, and with just a little clipping and maintenance, can be made into a low hedge, a knot or rock garden, or grown in containers. Bees and butterflies adore hyssop.

ABOUT HYSSOP

OTHER COMMON NAMES Hyssop doesn't have any regional nicknames that I could find.

SAFETY CONSIDERATIONS There are no known warnings for the plant; however, pregnant women and individuals with seizure disorders or with high blood pressure should avoid hyssop essential oil. Never take it internally.

PARTS USED all aerial parts

ENERGETICS warm, dry, spicy, slightly bitter

PROPERTIES Hyssop is antibiotic, antioxidant, anti-inflammatory, antispasmodic, antiviral, astringent, carminative, diaphoretic, expectorant, and nervine, and supports and stimulates the immune system.

USES Hyssop is used for sore throats, colds and congestion, hoarseness, coughs, and mild asthma. It can be helpful for urinary tract inflammations. It is good for the whole digestive system, assisting in appetite stimulation, colic, and excess gas. It calms nervousness and anxiety, and stops spasms of the lungs and gut. Hyssop has several illness-busting properties that

means it can fight viral infections and bacterial infections, and ease inflammation. It encourages perspiration to help break a fever. It is sometimes used externally on wounds and insect bites. Hyssop is revered in ritual and healing, and is well-known as a purifier physically, emotionally, and spiritually. You can burn hyssop to dispel negativity or make it into a cleansing tea. Although biblical scholars have determined that the hyssop mentioned in the Bible was most likely another plant, it is still revered in ritual and healing.

PREPARATIONS Tea is most commonly used, but tinctures and syrups are good to have on hand. Externally, poultices and compresses work well.

DOSAGE All preparations may be used several times daily as needed.

GROWING TIP Hyssop blooms from June through October and is generally considered to be evergreen. I like to dry some of it while it is in bloom each year, but there are almost always leaves out there in case of emergency. It is extremely easy to grow and a pretty little plant, too.

Home treatments

If you have gas and digestion problems, hyssop is a gentle remedy. The easiest method of delivery is as an ingredient in food. The aromatics and taste of hyssop can overpower delicate flavors, so experiment a bit and start with spare amounts. A little pre- or post-dinner tea is also comforting. Tincture and syrup are other options, but I prefer to start using an herb as food or drink whenever possible.

The warm, dry, and spicy energetics of hyssop are powerful for a cold that needs to dry up and move along. It's particularly helpful for those colds that seem to linger and bounce around like a ping-pong ball, going from head to chest and back again. Teas, tinctures, and syrups are all effective.

HYSSOP DEEP-CLEANSING MASK

Makes about 5 mask applications
Prep time: 15 minutes

The ingredients of this mask clean and freshen the skin while drawing impurities from the pores. It's good for any skin type and can be adjusted to be more astringent or more emollient by changing the liquid used. Oil or yogurt might be used for drier skin types, while witch hazel or black tea would act as astringents for more oily skin.

INGREDIENTS

2 tablespoons dried hyssop

2 teaspoons dried plantain

2 tablespoons ground kaolin or French green clay

2 teaspoons ground activated charcoal

SUPPLIES

a blender

coffee grinder, or mortar and pestle

a small jar

1. In a blender or coffee grinder, or using a mortar and pestle, grind the hyssop and plantain to a fine powder.

2. Transfer the powder to a bowl and mix in the kaolin and activated charcoal.

3. Place in a small jar and store until ready to use.

4. To use, choose your preferred base or liquid—you can use plain water, oil, rose water, plain yogurt, witch hazel, carrot or cucumber juice, or milk. (Anything liquid will probably work as long as it is skin-safe.) Mix 1 tablespoon of the powder mixture with enough of the base or liquid to make a thin, spreadable paste (the amount of base/liquid will vary greatly depending on what you use, but start with 1 teaspoon and keep adding until the desired thickness is reached). Spread the mask on your face, relax for 10 or 15 minutes, and rinse off.

HYSSOP TEA BLEND FOR COUGHS AND COLDS

Makes about 14 cups
Prep time: 15 minutes

This is a great tea to drink when you have gobs of wet, runny mucus. Between the hyssop and the yarrow, the tea will help you get more comfortable, and the elder blossoms step in to assist the hyssop in warming the body and inducing a sweat.

INGREDIENTS

½ cup dried hyssop

¼ cup dried elder blossoms

1 tablespoon dried yarrow

1 tablespoon dried peppermint

1 tablespoon dried ginger pieces

Honey, for serving (optional)

Lemon juice, for serving (optional)

SUPPLIES

a tea ball

In a bowl, mix together the hyssop, elder blossoms, yarrow, peppermint, and ginger. Place a heaping tablespoon of the blend into a tea ball and place in 1 cup of hot water. Cover and steep for 5 to 10 minutes. Drink as needed, using honey and lemon to taste if desired. The acid of the lemon helps cut through mucus during a wet cold, so use plenty.

Lavandula officinalis

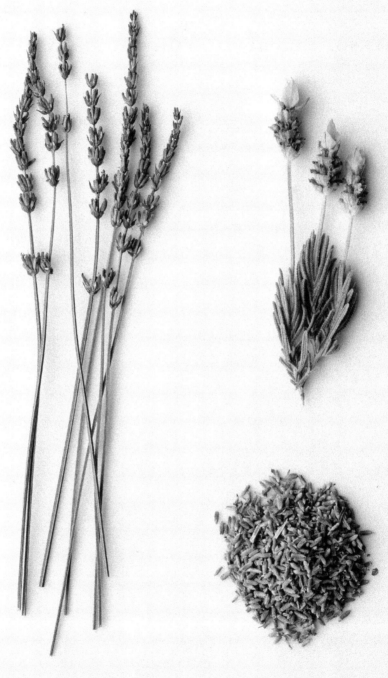

Lavender spp.

LAVENDER

Lavender is always in my garden. At first, I wasn't fond of the scent, but as I learned and experienced the benefits of this gorgeous herb, it quickly rose in my list of favorites. Native to the Mediterranean region, lavender has 30 to 50 different species and cultivars. Some are grown for beauty, some for culinary uses, some for the essential oil, and others for the scent. Lavender's name may have come from a couple different Latin derivations. The most popular theory is that it comes from *lavare*, which means "to wash," or it may come from *livere* meaning "bluish." Either works. Lavender has become hugely popular and is now available in hundreds of products, from household cleaners to candles, room sprays, essential oils, and desserts and candy. I prefer using the herb instead of the essential oil whenever possible.

ABOUT LAVENDER

OTHER COMMON NAMES Lavandula, English lavender, French lavender, garden lavender, spike lavender, sweet and true lavender

SAFETY CONSIDERATIONS There are no known precautions for the herb. However, overuse or undiluted use of the essential oil has been known to sensitize the user, which can be debilitating.

PARTS USED For essential oil, all aerial parts. In medicinal preparations, the unopened flower buds.

ENERGETICS cool and warming, toning and relaxing, pungent, bitter taste

PROPERTIES Lavender is a powerhouse of healing, with antibiotic, antidepressant, antifungal, anti-inflammatory, antiseptic, antispasmodic, antiviral, carminative, and aromatic properties. It is also relaxing and sedative.

USES The heady aromatics of the fresh or dried herb and the herbal constituents combine for a remedy that relaxes muscles and eases spasms that accompany muscular pain. A tea, tincture, or vinegar can help digestion, gas, nausea, and intestinal cramping. The herb in a sachet encourages sleep and helps with tension headaches. Topically, lavender tea, balm, or vinegar can help treat fungal infections, wounds, eczema, and varicose ulcers, soothe sunburned or windburned skin, heal burns, and calm acne. Lavender is a great herb for women's issues—it eases menstrual cramps, tension, and depression, and in menopause can help with insomnia.

PREPARATIONS tea, tincture, infused oil (used in all kinds of topical applications), vinegar, sachets for inhalation, and essential oil

DOSAGE Tea (equivalent of 1½ teaspoons lavender per cup of water) is safe to take up to three times a day. You can take 10 to 15 drops of tincture before meals for digestion or as needed up to three times a day, or 2 tablespoons of vinegar used in cooking per day. Dilute the essential oil to 10 drops per ounce of carrier oil.

GROWING TIP Depending on your growing zone, different species or cultivars will be hardy, although those in zones 5 or below may not be able to keep lavender outside over the winter. I like the long-stemmed, big spikes of the camphorous Grosso for weaving wands, but the English Munstead variety has a sweeter scent and taste.

Home treatments

Lavender is so cleansing, healing, and soothing that it's almost all-purpose. Inhaling the herb is surprisingly effective for headaches, restlessness, or anxiety. Once, at the renaissance festival, the king asked my sister and me for a headache remedy that would have been appropriate for the time. My sister did a little research overnight, and we returned with a little pillow filled with lavender and a few pinches of other herbs. It worked, and we had to make a lot of them, since he wandered around all summer sniffing it, and then everyone wanted one.

When my daughter was in second grade, she was an anxious child. I made her a very small stuffed cat filled with dried lavender, although a simple little pillow would have worked just the same. She loved it, and I've had to refill it a couple of times over the years, after the lavender inside was loved to dust.

LAVENDER POWDER

Makes 2 cups
Prep time: 10 minutes, plus at least 2 weeks to infuse

This powder has several benefits. Lavender is soothing to the skin, so there's the comfort factor. It is also calming and relaxing, and helps slow down perspiration that comes from stress. It can help decrease fungal or bacterial issues forming from damp areas and creases.

On top of all of this, it smells pleasant. You can increase the fragrance by adding 10 to 15 drops of lavender essential oils to the powder if desired.

INGREDIENTS

1 cup arrowroot powder

½ cup cornstarch

¼ cup kaolin or French green clay

¼ cup lavender, powdered in a blender or coffee grinder

SUPPLIES

a 1-quart jar

1. Blend together all of the ingredients in a 1-quart jar. The extra room makes it easy to shake often and be sure that everything is mixed well. Keep the mix in the jar for at least 2 weeks or up to a month for the scent to permeate the other powders, shaking it at least once every few days.

2. To use, pour a small amount of the powder into palm of your hand and smooth onto your body to remedy chafing or excessive perspiration.

TIP Powder shaker jars are available from suppliers listed in the Resources section (page 221), and they are perfect to use here; a wide-mouth jar with a powder puff works as well.

LAVENDER SACHET

Makes 1 sachet
Prep time: 15 minutes if using a muslin bag; 1 hour if making the bag from scratch

These simple sacks come in handy in innumerable ways. You can tuck them into drawers or closets, into your car to keep it smelling pleasant, in the bedside table to reach for during a restless night, or in a desk drawer or locker to pull out on bad days at work or school. Unless exposed to bright light and heat, dried lavender retains its scent until it turns to dust. If the scent fades, scrunch the sachet a few times to refresh it.

INGREDIENTS

1 cup dry lavender buds

SUPPLIES

1 piece of 9-by-6½-inch cloth or a 4-by-
   6-inch muslin bag
thread
needle

1. If using the cloth, fold it in half so that the right side is inside and the new size is 4½-by-6½ inches. Starting at the edge of the fold, using a needle and thread and a straight or running stitch (sewmyplace.com/project/tutorial-two-ways-to-make-a-simple-sachet is helpful), sew two sides together, leaving one of the 4½-inch sides open. Turn the cloth right-side out.

2. For cloth or the muslin bag, fill three-quarters of the way full, with about a cup of the lavender. Turn in the edges of the open end and sew shut.

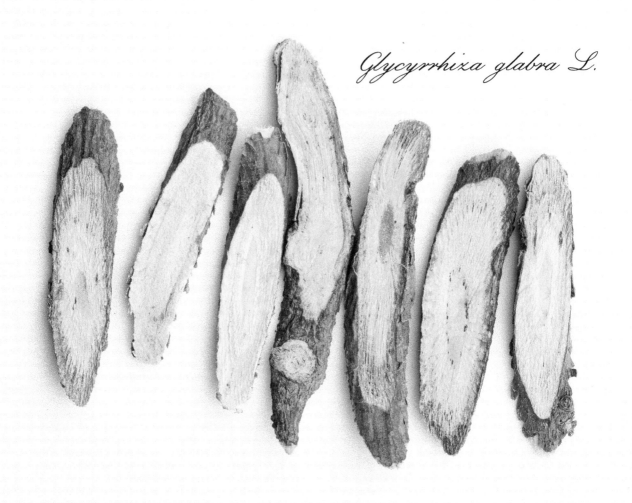

Glycyrrhiza glabra L.

LICORICE ROOT

Most of us think of licorice as a black, soft, and chewy candy that comes in jelly beans, "whips," and various other forms. Candy licorice pipes were at one time a popular shape, perhaps to signal to pipe smokers that it would calm smoker's cough. Licorice is very sweet, up to 50 times sweeter than sugar, making it an excellent ingredient for herbal tea. Although the licorice plant is native to southern Europe and Asia, northern European countries are absolutely obsessed with it and eat more licorice than chocolate. The Netherlands is a top licorice candy producer in the European Union. In the U.S., most licorice candy is flavored with anise, which isn't licorice at all, so it requires some hunting to find the real thing. Real licorice is made almost entirely from the licorice root.

ABOUT LICORICE ROOT

OTHER COMMON NAMES gan zao, sweet root, drop

SAFETY CONSIDERATIONS Avoid licorice in pregnancy. Individuals with high blood pressure, liver disorders, water retention, renal insufficiency, low blood potassium, or heart disease should also avoid this herb.

PART USED dried root

ENERGETICS sweet, cool, moisturizing

PROPERTIES Licorice root is adaptogenic, antibacterial, anticonvulsive, anti-inflammatory, antispasmodic, antiviral, demulcent, expectorant, immune-boosting, and laxative.

USES Licorice root is great for anyone trying to stop smoking. It satisfies that hand to mouth compulsion and provides a slight boost of energy, preventing the metabolism from getting sluggish as it so often does while quitting tobacco. Licorice promotes excretion of dry, stuck mucus, and can also ease bronchitis. It soothes gastrointestinal problems from mouth to anus, such as heartburn, GERD, ulcers, and constipation, and is considered helpful for adrenal fatigue. It's one of the most commonly used herbs in traditional Chinese medicine, as it is believed to guide other herbs to their best healing expression.

PREPARATIONS Licorice is useful as teas, tinctures, capsules, and pastilles. You can purchase licorice root as root sticks, cut and sifted, powdered, and as candy (just be sure the candy's made from licorice root and not anise flavoring). You can chew the licorice root sticks plain; they're also safe for children.

DOSAGE It's safe to drink up to 3 cups of licorice root tea or take 3 droppers of tincture per day. Be sure to pulse (stopping after about 10 days) rather than take daily for an extended period. Be aware that the candy is much more concentrated than the root.

TIP During cooler weather, when germs fly around, I use a licorice root stick in almost every medicinal tea I drink. Simply pop it in the mug and let it stand as the tea steeps. Even if you don't care for black licorice candy, try a cup of tea. It's delicious and so soothing!

Home treatments

During our renaissance festival days, nearly all the actors would strain their voices from the 8 or 10 hours of constant projection (some might say yelling). They'd come to our herb shop looking for help, so we always kept a healthy supply of licorice root sticks around. They effectively moistened and cooled sore throats, sending the actors back out there yelling . . . er, projecting, in no time.

A sore throat is often accompanied by hot, dry, and inflamed sinuses. The first sip of licorice tea brings nearly instant relief, soothing the parched mucus membrane. Licorice root brings similar relief for acid reflux. Plus, because you can just suck on the plain root, there's no need to drink anything that might exacerbate the situation. Licorice soothes the throat and sinuses where the acid has burned.

Constipation while traveling was an issue for my grandmother. She'd take me to the beach sometimes, and by about the second or third day, we'd have to go search for some real licorice candy. She always struggled with constipation when she was away from home. The demulcent property of licorice helps get things moving. Even better is a mug of hot licorice tea, since warm water is often helpful in digestion. I much prefer having the added liquid from the tea, since constipation is often partially brought on by dehydration in the system, causing hard, dry stools.

LICORICE TOOTH POLISH POWDER

Makes about ⅓ cup
Prep time: 15 minutes

The ingredients in this tooth polish help clean stains and promote gum health. If you like the taste of licorice, then you're in for a tasty treat while cleaning! It is difficult to get spices or roots into a nice powder, so it's best to purchase these ingredients already powdered.

INGREDIENTS

¼ cup kaolin or bentonite clay

1 tablespoon baking soda

2 teaspoons fine sea salt

2 teaspoons licorice root, powdered

1 teaspoon activated charcoal, powdered

1 teaspoon peppermint, powdered

½ teaspoon clove, powdered

½ teaspoon thyme, powdered

SUPPLIES

a large jar

a small jar or container

1. In a large jar, combine all the ingredients and shake to mix well.

2. Keep about 1 tablespoon of the polish mix in a small jar or container. Put a pinch of the mixture in the palm of your hand and pick it up with a wet toothbrush. Brush as you normally would and rinse well.

3. Keep the bulk of the mixture stored in the large jar (this way, if the small container gets wet, the whole batch won't be ruined). It will keep for 2 years.

TIP If you prefer a paste, melt 2½ to 3 tablespoons of coconut oil. Mix in a pinch of the polish mixture. Use a pea-size dollop on your toothbrush.

THROAT SPRAY

Makes 3 cups
*Prep time: 40 minutes, plus over-
night soaking*

This blend of soothing roots and bark
is very effective for sore throats or
for when the voice is scratchy or has
vanished from illness or overuse. One
or two sprays can provide immediate
relief that lasts a good while, and the
spray is safe to reuse often throughout
the day.

INGREDIENTS

1 quart water

1 tablespoon licorice root

1 tablespoon slippery elm bark

1 tablespoon marshmallow root

1 tablespoon grated fresh gingerroot

1 cup 195-proof alcohol (such as Everclear)

SUPPLIES

a large

a heavy saucepan with a lid

a few 2- or 4-ounce plastic spray bottles

1. Combine the water and herbs in a
   large, heavy saucepan. Cover with
   a lid and soak overnight.

2. The following day, boil everything together until the liquid is
   reduced by half (to about 2 cups).

3. Strain well to remove all the
   solids, then let the liquid cool
   completely.

4. Add the alcohol.

5. Pour into spray bottles and use as
   needed. (I like to make and label
   several small bottles.) Store at
   room temperature; the spray will
   keep for 10 years.

Tilia spp.

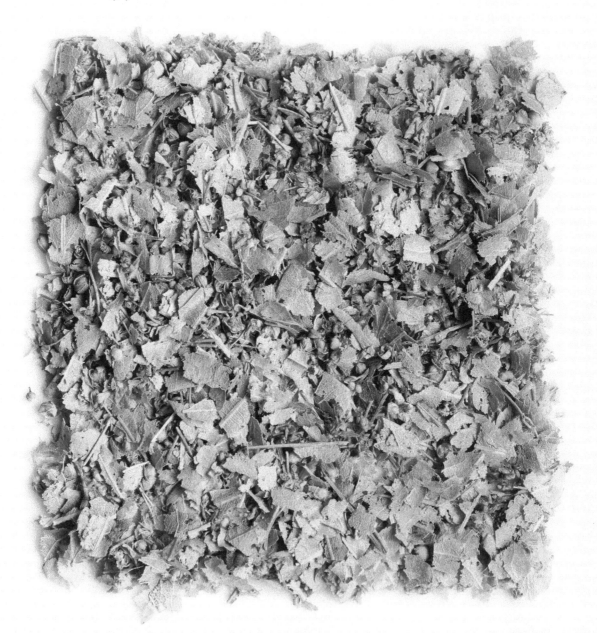

LINDEN

Linden is one of the most popular teas in Europe and the U.K. Given that it's such a common tree offering many benefits, it deserves to be better known in other locales as well. When I was just learning about linden, I found myself on a local 1700s homestead with an enormous old linden tree. It was alive with honeybees, and its fragrance filled the entire place. Down the farm lane and behind a barn, I found a tree with similar but larger flowers and leaves. I took a leaf and flower of each home and after a bit of research figured out that the small leaves come from a little-leaf linden, or *Tilia cordata*, while the large are from a big-leaf linden, or *Tilia platyphyllos*. These varieties are used interchangeably, and the little-leaf version is common in urban and suburban landscaping.

ABOUT LINDEN

OTHER COMMON NAMES Tilia, bass-wood, lime tree, lime flower

SAFETY CONSIDERATIONS Linden has been used safely since the Middle Ages. Excessive use has, in rare cases, been associated with heart damage in individuals with heart disease. If you have a heart condition, talk to your doctor before using.

PARTS USED the flowers with the attached leaf-like bract

ENERGETICS sweet, moisturizing, warm

PROPERTIES Linden is a nervine that is also demulcent, antibacterial, antifungal, antispasmodic, and astringent. It is highly valued for its sedative, expectorant, diaphoretic, and diuretic effects.

USES Since linden is a very common tree in temperate climates, it's a star player in folk medicine. Restlessness, insomnia, hyperactivity in children, nervous and muscle tension, anxiety, and headaches (especially migraines) all respond well to linden. The mucilage produced by the plant soothes digestive issues and may also help calm irritated membranes in the mouth or throat and decrease mucus production.

Linden also relieves muscle spasms and cramps and improves circulation. One of the most noted uses of linden is in inducing perspiration for feverish colds, flu, and infections. It also helps reduce nasal congestion and calm coughs. Externally, you can use linden as a wash or lotion for itchy skin. In an emotional sense, linden is often used for grief or heartache. In the doctrine of signatures, the heart-shaped leaves hint to this purpose. We can also look to linden's relaxing properties and sedative support of the nerves as assisting us through difficult, heartbreaking times.

PREPARATIONS Linden is easy to find or make as a tea. You can also make it into a tincture, syrup, or vinegar. Teas, tinctures, and vinegars can be used in topical preparations, such as a face wash or foot bath.

HARVESTING TIP Harvest linden in early summer, when the fragrant flowers are just beginning to bloom, picking the flowers along with the pale-green bract. While in bloom, the tree will most likely be buzzing with bees—they love linden and make a tasty honey from the flowers. Go slowly to avoid getting stung!

Home treatments

Linden tea brings relief in cases of cold or flu that includes dry, hacking coughs, swollen and inflamed air passageways, fever, and congestion. It can promote sleep and rest with its sedative properties, and has been known to relieve headaches. One day a friend and I were stuck working a long day in the herb shop and both of us felt something coming on. We brewed up some strong linden tea, and in no time at all we were both feeling a sweat coming on. We added some elderberry and holy basil and nipped that illness in the bud.

Linden is truly a friend during a period of insomnia brought about by grief or heartache. Once someone dear to me was stricken with a serious disease, and I wasn't able to see them in person for a long while. Needless to say, I was devastated. Linden tea helped me find some much-needed rest and sleep during this painful time.

LINDEN SYRUP

Makes about 2½ to 3 cups
Prep time: 30 minutes, plus overnight to steep

It's great to have this syrup handy and ready to use in case someone in your household starts feeling low, ill, or restless. It can be taken by the tablespoon as medicine, or used to flavor tea, sparkling water, or food. While this recipe uses linden flowers and bracts and traditional honey, you can find linden honey made from the flowers to mix with the water and lemon instead. Like maple, the linden tree's sap can be gathered and boiled down to a syrup, which would also work mixed with water and lemon.

INGREDIENTS

4 to 5 cups linden flowers and bracts

1½ cups water

3 cups honey

Juice of 1 lemon

SUPPLIES

a saucepan with a lid

bottles

1. Clean the linden flowers and bracts by giving them a good shake and a quick dunk in water. Strain in a colander and set aside.

2. Combine the water, honey, and lemon juice in a saucepan and simmer until thickened and reduced by about one-quarter.

3. Remove from the heat and add the flowers and bracts. Stir well and cover.

4. Let the syrup steep overnight, then strain out the solids and bottle the syrup. Store at room temperature and use within 1 year.

LINDEN AND PASSIONFLOWER ELIXIR

Makes about 16 ounces
Prep time: 15 minutes, plus 1 month to steep

I like to combine linden with passion-flower to help with sleeplessness. Passionflower is specifically helpful for those times when thoughts go around and around in your head. The two herbs used together have a calming and sedative effect.

INGREDIENTS

1½ cups brandy

½ cup honey

¾ cup dried linden

¾ cup dried passionflower

Zest and juice of 1 lemon

SUPPLIES

a 24-ounce jar

1. In a 24-ounce jar, combine the brandy and honey. Stir or shake until the honey is dissolved.

2. Add the linden, passionflower, and lemon zest and juice, and mix very well.

3. Allow everything to steep for at least 1 month, shaking daily if possible.

4. Strain out and discard the solids and use the elixir by the dropperful. You can also add a teaspoon to a cup of tea or a small glass of plain brandy.

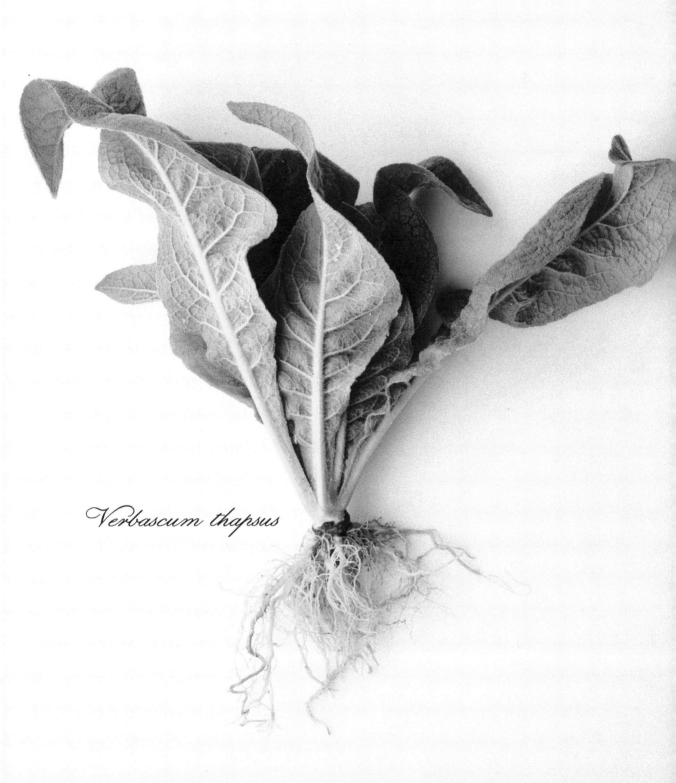

Verbascum thapsus

MULLEIN

Mullein was historically used in Africa, Greece, and parts of Europe before settlers brought it over to the Americas in the 1600s and it became part of the herbal healing tradition in the West. Native Americans quickly found plentiful medical uses for the plant. Mullein grows in rocky, dry, and disturbed soils, as well as in meadows or fencerows. It requires full sun and must have some cold weather in order to produce flower spikes in the second year. It has many healing benefits and is also an attractive enough plant to grow as an ornament in the garden.

ABOUT MULLEIN

OTHER COMMON NAMES great mullein, common mullein, candlewick plant, clown's lungwort, velvet dock, Quaker rouge, torchwort, hag's taper, flannel leaf, Aaron's rod, Jupiter's staff, St. Peter's staff, shepherd's staff, shepherd's club, beggar's stalk, golden rod, Adam's flannel, beggar's blanket

SAFETY CONSIDERATIONS The fine hairs on this plant can irritate skin and mucus membranes, so be sure to strain preparations well.

PARTS USED leaves, flowers, roots

ENERGETICS bitter, cool, moisturizing, salty

PROPERTIES Mullein is anodyne, antibacterial, anti-catarrhal, anti-inflammatory, antispasmodic, antitussive, antiviral, astringent, demulcent, diuretic, emollient, expectorant, nervine (mild), sedative, and also vulnerary. It's also a natural disinfectant.

USES The flowers and leaves are most often used. Both are mucilaginous, coating and soothing respiratory passages, clearing excess mucus from the airways and lungs, and soothing dry coughs. Mullein is useful as an antiviral and antibiotic, staving off illness. It also reduces inflammation of mucus membranes and calms muscle spasms while also relieving pain. It is used to prevent or relieve coughs and get rid of a tickle in the throat. Mullein is also good for joint pain, both applied externally and taken internally. The warm flower oil is useful for hemorrhoids. Mullein promotes healing of wounds, cuts, and abrasions, and, when infused and warmed with a little garlic, makes an effective ear drop for earaches and infections. The leaves have a long tradition as the main ingredient in smoking blends used for asthma and lingering coughs. It also helps urinary issues and increases urine output. It is thought to tone the bladder, support prostate health, and reduce inflammation of the urinary tract.

PREPARATIONS Teas, tinctures, infused oil, or poultices. The leaves can be smoked.

DOSAGE Mullein is considered nontoxic. It's safe to use as needed.

GROWING/HARVESTING TIPS The first-year plant is a basal rosette of fuzzy, pale blue-green leaves, and those are the roots to harvest for medicine. The second-year plant shoots up a stem topped with flowers. The leaves are always good to harvest. If you harvest the roots, be sure there are other plants around so you'll have more next year.

Home treatments

The mucilaginous property of mullein is exceptional for helping move a hot, dry cold up and out of the chest or to help drain the sinuses. Mullein has a special talent for moistening and loosening all the tight, tense areas of the upper-respiratory system and then relaxing the muscles and allowing mucus to flow freely in order to be coughed up. Hot mullein tea in a mug also allows inhalation of the steam, increasing these actions. Its mild sedative properties promote restful sleep.

Using mullein for hemorrhoids is very effective. The pain-reducing and wound-healing abilities combine with the astringent yet emollient properties, and are complemented by anti-inflammatory and antibacterial strengths, to boot. Apply a warm poultice several times a day for very painful cases. You can make wipes with infused oil and apply several times a day for relief before hemorrhoids get a foothold.

EAR OIL

Makes about 4 ounces (depending on how absorbent the herbs are)
Prep time: 1 hour 15 minutes (15 minutes active)

This is a time-tested remedy. Although it fell out of favor due to the use of pharmaceuticals, ear oil is becoming an herbal standard again. The warmed oil is soothing on its own, but the garlic and mullein work together to clear infection and inflammation.

INGREDIENTS

⅛ cup fresh or 1 tablespoon dried
   mullein flowers

3 tablespoons crushed garlic

¾ cup olive oil

SUPPLIES

an ovenproof 8-ounce (or larger) baking dish
   or ramekin

a jar

1. Place all the ingredients in an ovenproof 8-ounce (or slightly larger) baking dish or ramekin. Make sure everything is submerged in the olive oil, adding more oil if necessary.

2. Set the oven at the lowest possible setting (180°F to 200°F) and heat the oil for an hour. As an alternative, you can mix the ingredients in a jar and set in a warm, sunny window for a day.

3. Strain the oil thoroughly, transfer to a 4- to 6-ounce jar, and store in the refrigerator until needed. It will keep for a year.

4. To use, warm a small amount of the oil to about body temperature and place a few drops in the ear, rubbing the outside of the ear to distribute the oil and increase circulation. If tolerated, put a cotton ball in the ear to keep it warm, and rest the ear against a heating pad. Repeat as necessary every 30 to 60 minutes until the ear feels better.

SMOKING BLEND FOR STUBBORN CHEST COLD

Makes about ¼ cup
Prep time: 15 minutes

In terms of health, it's generally counterintuitive to smoke anything anymore. But sometimes there may be a therapeutic reason to do so. I've tried a few smoking blends for lung issues and have had great results with this one. Some people use blends to quit smoking. If they work and do no harm, you'll get no judgment from me there. Use freshly dried herbs in this recipe if possible (see Resources, page 221), or dry them yourself.

INGREDIENTS

3 tablespoons dried mullein leaf

1 tablespoon dried horehound

1½ teaspoons dried lavender

1 teaspoon dried peppermint

½ teaspoon dried California poppy (optional)

¼ teaspoon dried thyme (optional)

SUPPLIES

a coffee grinder

a pipe, rolling papers, or a vaporizer

1. Using a coffee grinder, grind all the herbs to similarly sized bits that are well blended. The mixture should have the consistency of tobacco.

2. Use a pipe, rolling papers, or a vaporizer to smoke, taking only one or two inhalations at a time.

Tropaeolum majus

Tropaeolum spp.

NASTURTIUM

Nasturtium is a perfect example of why it's important to know Latin names as well as the common names of plants. When you visit greenhouses and herb farms in spring to ask for nasturtium, you want to make sure you're getting the plans from the genus *Tropaeolum*, not *Nasturtium officinale*, which is actually watercress. The two plants share a spicy, hot flavor—and not much else. Nasturtium is native to South America and is mostly grown as an annual. The flowers come in shades from buttery yellow and creamy apricot to brilliant orange, red, and vibrant scarlet. In an informal taste test, my sister and I decided that the deeper the color, the spicier the flavor of the flower. It's in the leaves, however, where the medicinal properties reside.

ABOUT NASTURTIUM

OTHER COMMON NAMES Indian cress, garden nasturtium

SAFETY CONSIDERATIONS Pregnant women should avoid nasturtium. Additionally, it can cause contact dermatitis, so test a small area of skin before applying a poultice.

PARTS USED While the flowers are a delightful and delicious edible, and along with the leaves make a spicy addition to salads, the medicinal properties of the plant are found in the leaves prior to blooming. Some people eat the roots in the perennial varieties much like potatoes, but these aren't known to have medicinal properties . . . yet.

ENERGETICS hot, warming, dry

PROPERTIES Nasturtium leaves possess a surprising array of medicinal benefits. They are antibiotic, antibacterial, antifungal, antiseptic, antitussive, antiviral, diuretic, expectorant, and vulnerary, and a natural disinfectant.

USES Nasturtium tea has a long history of use in stimulating the scalp and encouraging healthy hair growth. It is used to help heal wounds, including those that show infection and are slow to heal. The leaves contain carotenoids and flavonoids, valuable compounds that boost the immune system, making nasturtium another great herb to fight against sore throats, coughs, bronchitis, congestion, and colds. Bacterial and fungal infections such as candida, ringworm, and athlete's foot respond well to soaking in nasturtium-leaf tea or applied poultices. Nasturtium also has the surprising ability to relieve symptoms of seasonal allergies, like sneezing, dry, itchy eyes, and runny nose, especially when combined with stinging nettle and local honey or bee pollen. The leaves and flowers are high in several B vitamins, vitamin C, and lots of minerals like iron, calcium, phosphorus, and manganese. It's been historically used for kidney problems and as a diuretic. For some, the tea helps with mild muscle pain.

PREPARATIONS Used in teas, tinctures, poultices, and as a wash, soak, or rinse

DOSAGE It's safe to drink the tea up to three times a day, take 25 drops of tincture three times a day, and use external applications as tolerated.

TIP Nasturtium seeds are very hot and spicy. They make a great little snack while working in the garden, or they can be grated and used like pepper or added to a spice blend for seasoning. We like to grind them with dried kelp, thyme, rosemary, and garlic to use at the table.

Home treatments

Nasturtium leaves mixed with Epsom salts make a splendid soak for sore, hot, tired feet, or as a bath tea to soothe skin abrasions, cuts, or strained muscles and rinse away dirt and sweat after a long day spent outside (think: gardening). This bath perks us up and fights fungus, germs, and grunge, and will also help wash off all the allergens that might come from a day in the garden and cause itchy eyes and sniffles. And while you're soaking away in there, have a nice hot cup of fresh nasturtium-leaf tea with some peppermint, rosemary, and stinging nettles, sweetened with local raw honey to help clear up those pesky allergy symptoms.

NASTURTIUM PESTO

Makes about 3 cups
Prep time: 20 minutes

How's this for a delicious medicine?
My favorite way to incorporate
healing herbs is by adding them to
scrumptious meals. Make this pesto
ahead and freeze into ½-cup portions
to be used as part of a yummy cam-
paign to prevent illness. Some people
don't add the cheese before freezing, and instead add it at the time of
serving, but I've never had a problem.
We use this pesto up pretty quickly in
my house.

INGREDIENTS

2 cups fresh nasturtium leaves

½ cup walnuts

6 garlic cloves

½ cup freshly grated Parmesan cheese

¾ cup olive oil

Hot sauce (optional)

SUPPLIES

a large saucepan

blender

resealable bags

1. Blanch the nasturtium leaves in
   a large saucepan of boiling water
   for 10 to 15 seconds. Drain and
   plunge the leaves into ice water to
   cool. Dry gently on tea towels.

2. Place the leaves, walnuts, garlic,
   cheese, and olive oil in a blender;
   blend until smooth. If desired,
   add a few drops of hot sauce.

3. Drizzle over pasta or the dish of
   your choice. Freeze in ¼-cup servings in resealable bags and use as
   desired within 3 to 4 months.

NASTURTIUM TINCTURE (OR HAIR RINSE)

Makes 1 pint
Prep time: 15 minutes, plus about 1 month to steep

As pointed out above, nasturtium leaves are the most potent part of the plant before it blooms. This tincture does a good job of preserving the healing properties of those early leaves. Take 1 teaspoon of the tincture up to three times a day. To make this recipe as a hair rinse, use vinegar instead of alcohol. The hair rinse is thought to promote hair growth by keeping the scalp healthy and stimulated—pour about ½ cup on the hair immediately after washing, massage in thoroughly, then rinse.

INGREDIENTS

1 cup fresh nasturtium leaves

¼ cup rosemary needles

¼ cup stinging nettle leaves

2 cups 100-proof vodka (or apple cider vinegar for the hair rinse)

SUPPLIES

a 1-pint jar

1. Place all the herbs in a pint jar and cover with the vodka (or apple cider vinegar if making hair rinse).

2. Cover and let the mixture steep in a cool, dry place for about 1 month. Check that the herbs are submerged in the liquid a couple of times a day, shaking the jar as necessary to ensure that the herbs are completely saturated.

3. After about a month, run the mixture through a food processor and strain well. Both the tincture and the rinse will last indefinitely at room temperature.

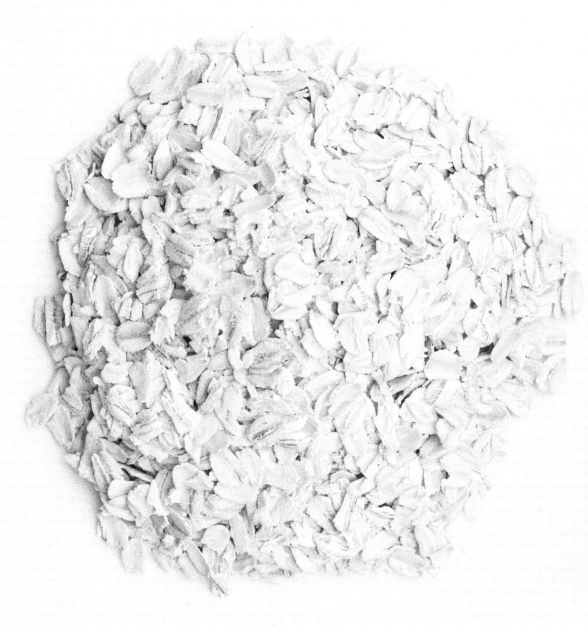

Avena sativa

OATS

Most people generally don't think about oats as an herb. It's a good, hearty breakfast food and an ingredient in cookies or granola bars, and is sometimes added to broths and meatloaf, right? But wild oats have plenty of medicinal benefits. They are rampant in my yard, planted regularly by birds, I assume. They're a type of grass, with the grain being the seed. It's possible to purchase oat seeds that produce larger grains, but the wild ones work for me. Each year I leave a couple of patches until they've gotten to the right stage, and then I harvest them and reclaim the bit of land they were on for other plants.

ABOUT OATS

OTHER COMMON NAMES wild oats, common oats, oatstraw

SAFETY CONSIDERATIONS None—oats are considered to be safe.

PARTS USED all aerial parts

ENERGETICS sweet, warming, relaxing, moisturizing

PROPERTIES Oats are a restorative, nutritive, and nervine tonic that slowly build up our resilience. They're also an antidepressant.

USES Oats are wonderful and skin-soothing when used in bathwater. In the bath section, I mentioned how my mom used to fill the kitchen sink with warm water, oatmeal, and me, and how I used the same treatment with my daughter. The water turns silky and a little milky, soaking away itches and irritation, and moisturizing the skin. This is essentially how aerial parts of the oat plant work internally, too. When the whole plant is harvested and dried while green, including the seeds, it is called oatstraw. Oatstraw is a rejuvenating and restorative nourishing mineral tonic. Milky oats are the most commonly discussed form of oats. For just a few days, the unripe seeds excrete white, milky latex when squeezed. This latex, particularly when used fresh, is a super nerve tonic that feeds and strengthens the nerves and their communication pathways. Milky oat tincture is the best way to access the herb's potential, and helps with adrenal exhaustion, difficulty concentrating, loss of libido, anxiety, depression, irritability, and postpartum blues. It is grounding, helping fortify us during grief, and promotes emotional well-being. Oatmeal is the ripe seed. It nourishes and lubricates throughout the body and the skin while supporting the nervous system.

PREPARATIONS teas, tinctures, in baths and on the skin, and in food

DOSAGE Teas and tinctures can be taken several times daily. Use externally as needed.

HARVESTING TIP The trickiest thing about the milky oat stage is catching it at the right time. When the kernels begin to develop, be sure you have your alcohol ready to go in the house because it is only milky for about a week. Test for the milk (latex) every day by pinching one of the oats. When a small drop of white liquid appears, it is time to make tincture. There won't be another chance until next year.

Home treatments

Oats work wonders for adults who are stretched to the limits with stressful jobs, young children, aging parents, and not enough hours in the day. More often than not, a little grounding comes in handy, and a daily dose of milky oat tincture fits that bill.

Oatmeal as a regular part of your diet is filling and soothing to the nerves, and its fiber and bulk contribute to regularity. Oats are a very simple "herb" to add to daily life.

BLUE OAT SMOOTHIE

Makes two 12-ounce servings
Prep time: 15 minutes

This meal-in-a-glass will help support the nerves and the immune system all day long. I like to add blueberries for their anthocyanins, and the addition of the holy basil and astragalus add to the adaptogenic power of this blend. You can also add different herbs and spices, such as some ginger, rose, nettles, or a pinch of lavender.

INGREDIENTS

½ cup old-fashioned rolled oats

1 cup milk (any kind)

½ cup frozen blueberries

2 tablespoons honey

1 small banana

½ cup ice

1 teaspoon dried holy basil

½ teaspoon powdered astragalus

SUPPLIES

a blender

1. Put all the ingredients in a blender. Cover tightly and pulse to break up the ice cubes.

2. Continue pulsing until smooth. Check consistency and add more milk if necessary.

3. Serve immediately.

MILKY OAT TINCTURE

Makes about 2 cups
*Prep time: 15 minutes, plus 4 to 6
weeks to steep*

Milky oats make an unusual tincture in that the texture is thicker than that of most tinctures. This is totally normal, and you'll get used to it—trust me. After the healing properties are pulled into the alcohol, the steeping tincture will look almost gruel-like. Use a dropper or two a day.

INGREDIENTS

1½ cups fresh milky oats

2½ cups 151-proof alcohol (such as
   Everclear)

SUPPLIES

a blender

a large jar

1. Place the oats and alcohol in a blender and whirl together until the mixture reaches a slushy consistency; add more alcohol if necessary to achieve this consistency.

2. Transfer the mixture to a large jar and let steep for 4 to 6 weeks.

3. After 4 to 6 weeks, strain the mixture well using a tincture press or by spooning it into a muslin bag and squeezing.

4. Store the tincture in the large jar at room temperature. It will keep for more than 10 years.

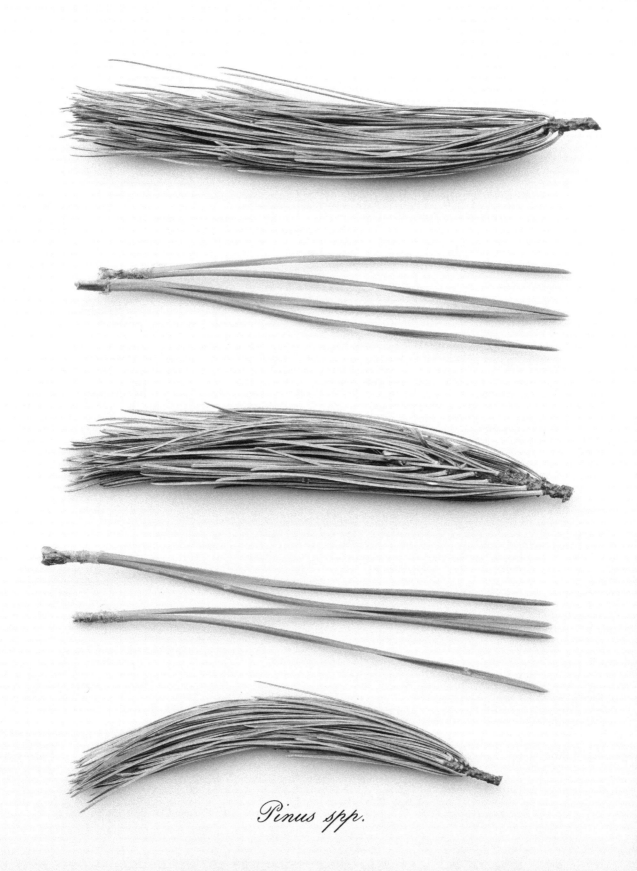

Pinus spp.

PINE

I live on the edge of a Christmas tree farm,
so it seemed only right to include pine in
the lineup of herbs for this book. All pines
are conifers, but there are many conifers
that are not pines. There are more than
30 kinds of pine in North America and
125 worldwide. It's interesting to note
that there are more than 500 conifer
(cone-bearing) species in the world. Trees
like larch, spruce, cedar, and fir are conifers
but not pines. The most common pines
grow needles in bundles of two to five,
wrapped at the base by a paper-thin, shallow sheath where they attach to
the twig. It's important to identify the
trees properly. A good field guide will help
identify evergreens so you can use them
with confidence.

ABOUT PINE

OTHER COMMON NAMES Christmas tree, evergreen, tannenbaum

SAFETY CONSIDERATIONS Pine pollen can cause allergic reactions even in those who aren't normally allergic to pine. I found this to be true the first time I gathered it.

PARTS USED needles, pollen, and pitch/sap

ENERGETICS warm, dry

PROPERTIES The ubiquitous pine tree has a surprising number of benefits. The needles and sap are anodyne, anti-fungal, antibacterial, antiseptic, aromatic, astringent, anti-inflammatory, antioxidant, decongestant, expectorant, stimulant, and tonic. The pollen is nutritious enough to be considered a superfood; it's jam-packed with vitamins and has all nine essential amino acids. Taken regularly, it is thought to build and increase vitality.

USES The needles and sap are best known for treating upper-respiratory infections by penetrating and clearing mucus. Often the sap or essential oil is made into a chest rub that makes it easier for someone with a clogged head to breathe while loosening up the chest at the same time. Pine eases inflammation and swelling of the upper- and lower-respiratory systems. We use pine cleaners in our home, and the infusion of pine needle or sap in alcohol is a good disinfectant for wounds on skin, tissues, and membranes. Clearing away bacteria and all kinds of pathogens, pine speeds healing both inside and out.

Pine teas and tinctures of needles or sap are thought to improve circulation and boost immunity. Salves made from the sap can be used on muscle and joint pain, and the inner bark can be made into a field dressing to keep wounds clean and germ-free. Above all, a cup of pine tea just brings on that bright-eyed and bushy-tailed feeling, especially with an added pinch of peppermint and a spot of honey.

PREPARATIONS teas, tinctures, infused honey, infused oil, liniments, and salves

DOSAGE Pine teas, infused honey, and tinctures can be used up to three times a day. Externally, you can use a salve or infused oil as needed.

HARVESTING TIP Gathering pine sap is dirty work. Be sure to wear clothes that you don't mind getting ruined. Take a sharp knife and a small wax paper–lined tin. Look for globs of sap where the bark has been injured, and peel off and place into your tin. You can also find small pearls of sap inside the dropped cones.

Home treatments

The mild scent of pine provided by pine needle tea is invigorating and can sharpen cognitive powers. Personally, I find that pine perks up my spirits. In addition to drinking the tea, I carry a small vial of a combination of saps from different pine trees in my purse to sniff when I need to clear my head.

Pine sap salve is a good choice for feet and ankles where a lack of circulation may lead to ulceration of the skin. The warming, dry nature of pine relieves the cold and damp effects of too little exercise and retained water in the joints.

SAP INFUSION IN OIL OR TINCTURE

Makes about ¾ cup
Prep time for oil: 15 minutes,
plus 2 to 4 hours to steep on stove or
up to 1 month to steep in jar

Prep time for tincture: 15 minutes,
plus up to 1 month steeping

Make one or both of these ahead so
they are ready whenever you need
them! You can use the oil internally
as is, or make it into a healing and
warming salve. The aromatic properties of pine are an added bonus with
every use.

FOR THE OIL

¼ cup pine sap

½ cup olive oil or other oil of your choice

FOR THE TINCTURE

¼ cup pine sap

½ cup 190-proof (95 percent) alcohol
  (151-proof will also work)

SUPPLIES

an 8- or 12-ounce jar

TO MAKE THE OIL

1. Combine the pine sap and olive
   oil in an 8- or 12-ounce jar.

2. Place the jar in a warm place,
   such as a windowsill, and let steep
   for up to a month, shaking the jar
   daily if possible. Alternatively, if
   you're in a hurry, you can warm it
   in a double boiler for 2 to 4 hours,
   or until the sap is completely dissolved into the oil.

3. Strain well, bottle, and use as
   needed. The oil usually lasts at
   room temperature for a year
   or more.

TO MAKE THE TINCTURE

1. Combine the pine sap and alcohol
   in an 8- or 12-ounce jar.

2. Place the jar in a warm place,
   such as a windowsill, and let steep
   for up to a month, shaking the jar
   daily if possible.

3. Strain well, bottle, and use as
   needed. The tincture will last at
   room temperature for at least
   10 years.

PINE NEEDLE TEA

Makes 2 cups
Prep time: 15 minutes

Be sure to make this tea with fresh
or frozen-from-fresh pine needles.
Dried needles lose their vibrancy
very quickly. The flavor of the tea
is not as strong as you might think.
Some people love the flavor as is,
but I like to add something else like
hibiscus, peppermint, or lemon—and
always honey!

INGREDIENTS

2¼ cups water

½ cup pine needles, cleaned and cut into
  ½-inch pieces

SUPPLIES

a small saucepan with a lid

1. In a small saucepan, bring water
   to a boil.

2. Add the pine needles to the
   boiling water and remove from
   the heat.

3. Cover and let steep for 3 to
   5 minutes.

4. Strain and serve.

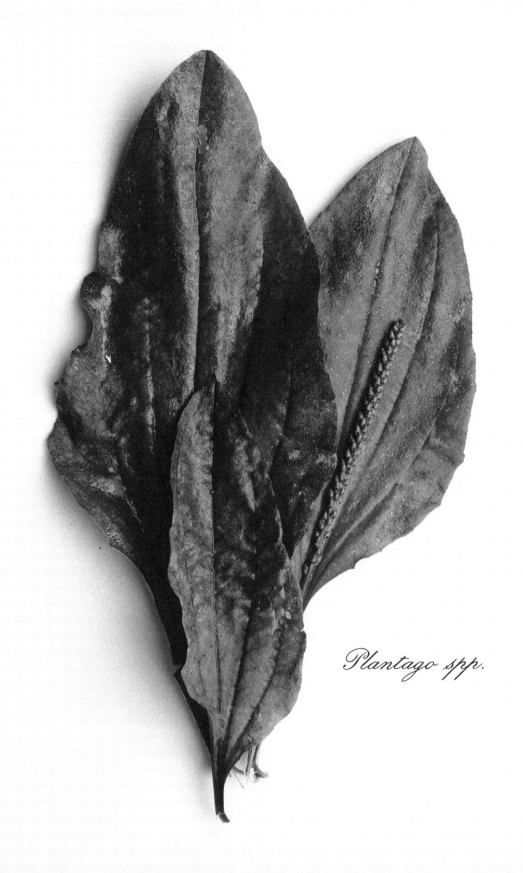

Plantago spp.

PLANTAIN

Plantain is the first "weedy" herb that most of us use. Not to be confused with the mild cooking bananas, this plant grows in a basal rosette, sending up slim seed stalks from the center. The leaves of the two most common species (*major* and *lanceolata*) in most of the U.S. have ribs all the way from the stem to the leaf tip. Plantain grows so abundantly in this country (and on nearly every continent) that there has never been a time when I needed it and couldn't find it, unless it was the deepest part of winter. I've even found it in midtown Manhattan, growing in sidewalk cracks! With a little planning, plantain is always there for us.

ABOUT PLANTAIN

OTHER COMMON NAMES rabbit ears, ribwort, waybread, waybroad, wagbread, whiteman's-foot, Englishman's-foot, cuckoo's bread, snakeweed, devil's shoestring, common plantain, ripple grass, healing blade, dooryard plantain, bird seed, rat-tail

SAFETY CONSIDERATIONS Plantains are completely safe for everyone, including infants and the elderly.

PARTS USED leaves, seeds

ENERGETICS salty, bitter, cool, moisturizing

PROPERTIES Plantain is alterative, analgesic, anti-inflammatory, antimicrobial, antispasmodic, astringent, decongestant, demulcent, diuretic, drawing, expectorant, refrigerant, tonic, and vulnerary.

USES Plantain is a whole medicine chest growing out of the ground. It contains allantoin and mucilage to speed healing of wounds, and vitamin K, which is essential to proper blood clotting. As an astringent, it clears up boggy areas and excess secretions in all areas of the body. The mucilage soothes and moistens membranes and tissues. Plantain is healing to the entire digestive system, beginning as a soothing gargle for mouth and gum irritations, then moving through the throat to calm soreness and into the esophagus where it can help relieve and soothe membranes that have been irritated with acid, and then into the stomach, where it is helpful in the case of ulcers. In the end (pun intended), it goes on to soothe the entire system and relieve constipation, bladder inflammation, hemorrhoids, and even the kidneys. *Psyllium* is a specific variety of plantain whose seeds are used specifically for digestion and regularity, but *major* and *lanceolata* will provide the desired mucilage. That same combination of astringency and mucilage is a boon for the respiratory tract, helping tighten, dry, and soothe. For the skin, it tackles insect bites, rashes, splinters, eczema, burns, and psoriasis.

PREPARATIONS teas, tinctures, salves, poultices, soaks, oils, vinegars, tub teas, face masks, and spit poultices

DOSAGE Plantain is considered very safe. You can use teas or tinctures up to three times daily. External use is safe to repeat as needed.

HARVESTING TIP Gather plantain leaves midday, when they are free of dew. Immediately process most of it either as a tincture or an oil infusion. I like to dry some to use during winter in teas or soups. This is one plant that you can gather without worrying about taking too much!

Home treatments

Plantain's drawing ability is remarkable on splinters and bee or wasp stings. I've even used it successfully on a blocked salivary gland. Poultices are most effective for this purpose, but compresses with warm tea or infused oil will also do the trick. A stubborn splinter straight that went into the pad of my thumb came right out with plantain, and the infection and pus came out along with it. Plantain is also very good for weepy rashes, like poison ivy. The astringent tannins dry up the fluid in the blisters and soothe and protect the skin at the same time. Plantain tea or tincture is good for someone with an overly dry constitution, as it will add some moisture and lubrication throughout the body in the organs and joints.

GARDEN AND WEED TEA

Yield varies based on amount of each ingredient used
Prep time: 15 minutes, plus gathering and drying time

I particularly enjoy gathering this tea blend with children or people who are new to herbs. You can add many different wild herbs, but those listed below have soothing, emollient, or relaxing properties. The exact amount of each ingredient doesn't matter too much. This is a forager's tea, and it is extremely flexible. If you're unable to forage, you can purchase all of the ingredients needed. Note that lavender and licorice have strong flavors that can overpower a blend, so use those ingredients sparingly.

INGREDIENTS

Plantain leaves

Marshmallow leaves and flowers

Violet leaves and flowers

Rose petals

Calendula flowers

Lemon balm or verbena leaves

Raspberry leaves

1 pinch licorice root

1 pinch lavender buds

SUPPLIES

a jar and a tea ball

1. The ingredients can be gathered in any amount. Try starting with a ¼ cup of each when fresh. Scatter the herbs on a screen and allow to dry—this can take 3 days to a week.

2. Once the herbs are dried, mix all of them together and keep the tea blend in a jar.

3. Add about 2 teaspoons of the tea blend to a tea ball. Put the tea ball in a mug, pour in hot water, and let steep for at least 5 minutes or up to 15 minutes.

PLANTAIN SALVE

Makes slightly more than 4 ounces
Prep time: 10 minutes

Keep this salve handy for all kinds
of household issues. You can put
it on burns (after the skin has
thoroughly cooled), splinters,
blemishes, or anywhere a drawing
salve is needed. It should have a
noticeable effect pretty quickly.
If it doesn't, switch to a poultice
without oil.

INGREDIENTS

4 ounces plantain-infused olive oil (or oil of
   your choice)

½ ounce beeswax

SUPPLIES

a double boiler

a few small glass jars

1. Heat the olive oil and beeswax
   gently in a double boiler until the
   wax has completely melted and
   combined with the oil.

2. Pour the salve into small jars.
   It will keep for 6 months at room
   temperature or for a year in the
   refrigerator. You'll know it's no
   longer good if the oil smells "off."

TIP You can also make this into an all-purpose salve by adding things like oils infused
with calendula, yarrow, St. John's wort, or
lavender.

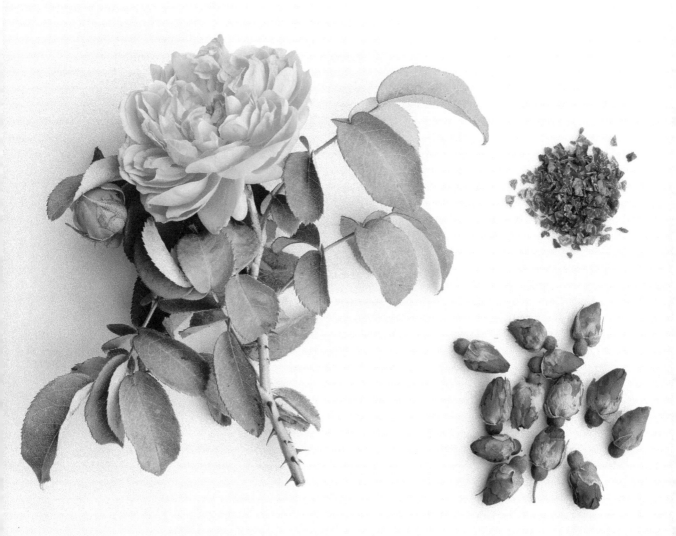

Rosa spp.

ROSE

The rose petal is soft and silky but very strong. It's very difficult to powder. Even crispy-dry, it doesn't crumble like other dried herbs. There are lots of documented physical benefits and uses for rose, but the more we get to know it, the more we understand the important benefits centered around our emotions. Rose is always considered the flower of love and gets trotted out every Valentine's Day, but it lives up to that name in ways we don't typically consider. Herbalists request remedies made from rose to support those who are facing trauma or disaster. The call is always "More rose! We need more rose!" Consider planting a rosebush for beauty and health.

ABOUT ROSE

OTHER COMMON NAMES apothecary rose, beach rose, briar hip, briar rose, cabbage rose, damask rose, dogberry, dog rose, eglantine gall, French rose, hep tree, hip fruit, hop fruit, hogseed, multiflora rose, rose hip, sweet briar, witches' briar, wild rose

SAFETY CONSIDERATIONS There are no official warnings for rose except for potential allergies. Rose hips have small hairs inside the seed capsule, so avoid piercing that. Strain well if used for tea.

PARTS USED whole flowers, petals, rose hips

ENERGETICS cooling, moisturizing, sweet

PROPERTIES Rose is analgesic, antianxiety, antibacterial, anti-inflammatory, antiseptic, antispasmodic, antiviral, aphrodisiac, astringent, calming, expectorant, nervine, nourishing, refrigerant, sedative, styptic, and tonic. A natural antidepressant, rose is used to combat grief and open the heart to feel joy.

USES Rose reduces the pain, heat, and inflammation of burns (especially sunburn), wounds, scratches, abrasions, rashes, bites, and stings. Rose tincture quickly calms the system during any kind of upset, particularly in the case of trauma, like an accident or unexpected shock. It is believed to benefit cardiac health and blood pressure, and improve poor circulation. Rose infusion strengthens bones and supports the endocrine system, helping women maintain regular menstruation and increasing fertility in men. Rose is also used for sore throats and mouth sores due to its astringency and moisturizing ability.

PREPARATIONS teas, tinctures, oils, infused honey, vinegars, flower essences, rose water, essential oils, soaps, poultices, compresses, and lotions

DOSAGE Teas and tinctures are safe to use as desired. Use the flower essence in 5- to 10-drop doses. Rose for external use is very gentle and safe.

TIP Fresh roses from florists are almost without fragrance, and they're typically grown with pesticides and preservatives. Grow your own or gather them in the wild. Once you've stuck your face in a basket of fresh wild or homegrown rose petals, there will be no going back to anything less.

Home treatments

Rose petal vinegar is great for sunburn or windburn, and is simple to make. Just infuse vinegar with piles of rose petals and allow it to steep until needed. Pour a cup or two of the vinegar into a warm bath and soak those raw edges away.

Rose has a long history of use for beauty. It is considered to be one of the premier ingredients to care for dry, sensitive, or aging skin. It's a natural toner that soothes and helps skin retain moisture. Ancient Egyptians used oils infused with roses to protect their skin from the dry winds of the desert. There are many ways to treat your skin to rose's benefits. My mother always loved glycerin and rose water (in a 50:50 ratio), but I prefer to just use rose water in a spray bottle. Other terrific options are to soak fresh rose petals in witch hazel for a spectacular toner; add rose petals to the bath; and infuse jojoba or apricot kernel oil with rose petals for a simple moisturizer.

ROSE AND RASPBERRY JAM

Makes about 3½ cups
Prep time: 1 hour

In this jam, the flavor and scent of the roses combine with the raspberries in an almost magical way. Plus, the raspberries contain pectin, so there's no need to add any. The deep, dark berries add antioxidants to all the great benefits of the roses. Spread this jam on your English muffin in the morning to start your day off right.

INGREDIENTS

1½ cups water

2 cups rose petals

1 cup black raspberries

2 cups sugar

1 tablespoon freshly squeezed
   lemon juice

SUPPLIES

a food processor

a medium saucepan

a few sterilized glass jars

1. Place the water and rose petals in a food processor and pulse to chop the petals into smaller pieces.

2. Pour the mixture into a medium saucepan and add the berries. Bring to a boil over high heat, then reduce the heat to low and simmer for 10 minutes.

3. Add the sugar and lemon juice, stirring to dissolve the sugar.

4. Simmer for another 20 to 30 minutes.

5. Remove from the heat and pour into hot sterilized jars.

6. Store the jam in the refrigerator for 2 to 3 months.

ROSE 'N' HERB COUGH SYRUP

Makes about 1 quart
Prep time: 1 hour

This syrup is yummy and effective. All of the herbs work together to moisten, tone, and soothe the throat and upper respiratory system. Even the little ones in the house will happily take this syrup.

INGREDIENTS

2 cups rose petals

½ cup peppermint

¼ cup plantain

2 tablespoons sage leaves

2 tablespoons mullein flowers

4 cups water

1½ cups sugar

½ cup honey

SUPPLIES

a food processor

a 2-quart saucepan

a few bottles

1. Combine the rose petals, peppermint, plantain, sage leaves, mullein flowers, and water in a food processor, and process to form a very thin slush.

2. Place the mixture into a 2-quart saucepan. Cover the pan and bring to a boil over high heat. Reduce the heat to low and simmer for 15 minutes.

3. Remove from the heat. Strain the liquid well.

4. Return the liquid to the pan and bring to a boil.

5. Add the sugar and stir until it is completely dissolved. Bring to a boil for 3 to 5 minutes. The mixture should begin to thicken.

6. Add the honey.

7. Let cool slightly and pour into bottles. The syrup will keep for up to a year in the refrigerator.

TIP I like to add a cup of brandy to the syrup to help preserve it longer (about 2 years), and for its added warming effect.

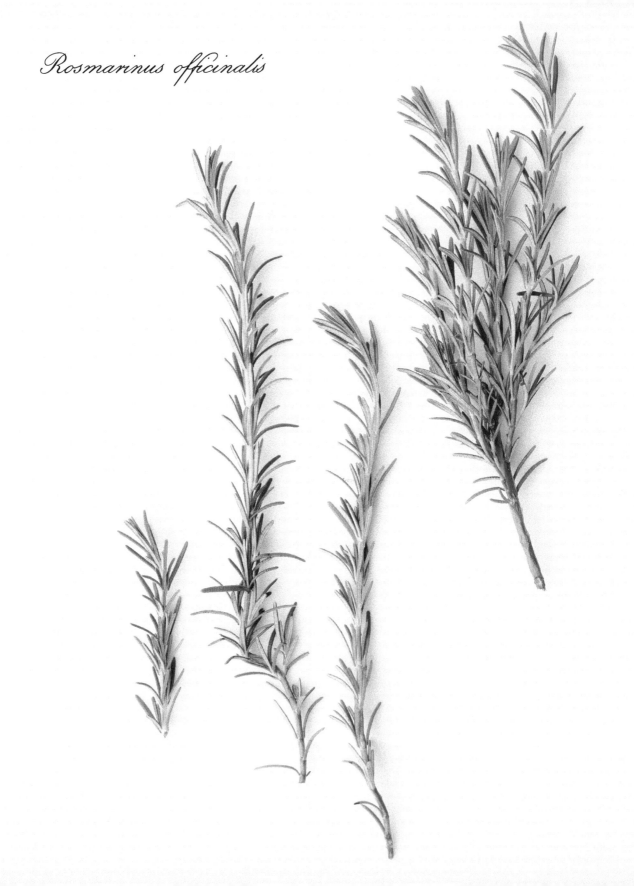

Rosmarinus officinalis

ROSEMARY

Rosemary comes with its share of herb lore, including tales of scholars wearing chaplets of rosemary about their heads to improve cerebral powers. Legend has it that the Virgin Mary draped her blue cloak over a rosemary shrub, turning the white flowers forever blue. Rosemary symbolizes remembrance and has a rich history in both weddings and funerals. Of course the fairies love rosemary and sometimes disguise themselves as snakes to hide beneath its branches. Sprigs or sachets of rosemary hung by the door are believed to protect the house and keep negativity away. And, of course, rosemary has many medicinal benefits.

ABOUT ROSEMARY

OTHER COMMON NAMES dew of the sea, old man, compass weed, compass plant

SAFETY CONSIDERATIONS Though rosemary is safe in moderation, large doses (particularly ingestion of the essential oil) may cause vomiting, seizures, pulmonary edema, uterine bleeding, and miscarriage. Rosemary can also interfere with some medications, such as anticoagulants, blood pressure medications, and diuretics.

PARTS USED stems, leaves, flowers

ENERGETICS warming, dry, pungent

PROPERTIES Rosemary is analgesic, antibacterial, antifungal, anti-inflammatory, antioxidant, antiseptic, antispasmodic, antiviral, aromatic, carminative, choleric, digestive, diuretic, nervine, neuroprotective, stimulant, tonic, and vulnerary. It is also a mild laxative and diuretic, stimulates menstrual flow, boosts the immune system, and may alleviate rheumatoid arthritis.

USES Rosemary is invigorating and fights exhaustion, weakness, and mild depression. It's stimulating without depleting energy. Teas and infused oils or vinegars can improve digestion, easing stomach cramping and excess gas. Rosemary is used externally on the scalp for dandruff and to stimulate hair growth, and also helps with eczema. Rosemary tea is great for circulation and memory, and is believed to slow down damage from degenerative joint disease. Rosemary is rich in antioxidants, which protect vision and skin, slow the effects of aging, and may protect cells from cancer. Research has been going on for decades around the effects of rosemary aromatherapy on cognitive abilities. The general consensus seems to be that a little fragrance is more beneficial than a lot, and rosemary does help with concentration and memory, especially in aging.

PREPARATIONS Teas, tinctures, infused oils and vinegars, soaps, essential oils, and sprays. It's commonly used, either fresh or dried, in cooking.

DOSAGE Using rosemary in food is generally safe in any quantity. When it comes to a tea or tincture, take no more than two doses daily when needed.

HARVESTING TIP In many parts of the world, including the southern and western parts of the U.S., rosemary grows in huge drifts and hedges. In my zone-6b location, it sometimes makes it through the winter and sometimes does not. To be safe, I harvest to just above the woody section of the stems every year. If it dies, it is easy to replace in the spring.

Home treatments

Years ago, a gastroenterologist scoffed when I mentioned that my digestive system felt slower than it should. My "normal" was indigestion, acid reflux, cramping, bloating, and constipation. Instead of pushing for the tests that she thought were a waste of time, I started eating more raw food and included rosemary tea in my diet at least a few times a week. Rosemary warms and stimulates movement throughout the stomach, intestines, and bowel. It took some time and was due to a combination of things, but eventually my problems disappeared.

Rosemary is the perfect herb for stress headaches. It contains salicylate that acts much like aspirin does on pain, muscle tension, and the like. It's also a good nervine and anti-inflammatory. Pain, stress, and inflammation often come together into something like a snowball rolling down a hill, growing with each turn. Rosemary can work against all three, bringing the sun out to melt that snowball.

ROSEMARY AND NETTLE HAIR AND SCALP RINSE

Makes about 1 quart (about 8 uses depending on length of hair)
Prep time: 10 minutes, plus 3 weeks to steep (or 4 to 6 hours in a slow cooker)

The vinegar in this rinse brings added protection around the hair cuticle. The rosemary and nettle are stimulating and strengthening, leaving the hair shiny and the scalp healthy.

INGREDIENTS

1 quart apple cider vinegar

1 cup fresh or ⅓ cup dried rosemary

1 cup fresh or ⅓ cup dried nettles

SUPPLIES

a large jar

a slow cooker (optional)

1. Combine all the ingredients in a large jar. Let steep at room temperature for 3 weeks. Alternatively, you can combine everything in a slow cooker and steep for 4 to 6 hours on low.

2. After steeping, strain well, pressing as much of the vinegar out of the herbs as possible.

3. Store in the jar at room temperature and use within a year.

4. To use, after washing hair, work ½ cup of the rinse (for medium-length) through hair and into the scalp. Rinse well. Any vinegar smell will vanish as hair dries.

SIMMERING POTPOURRI

Makes 6 or 7 simmers (each can be used at least twice)
Prep time: 15 minutes

This potpourri is especially useful in the winter when the air is drier. The steam combined with the aromatic, cleansing, and health-boosting properties of these herbs make this more than your average air freshener. This is an all-natural, gentle remedy for dry air in the home, and it smells amazing!

INGREDIENTS

½ cup dried rosemary needles

½ cup dried eucalyptus leaves

½ cup dried lavender buds

¼ cup dried orange or grapefruit zest

2 tablespoons dried gingerroot pieces

SUPPLIES

a pint jar

a small pot

1. Mix all the ingredients together in a pint jar.

2. To use, fill a small pot with water, and add about ¼ cup of the blend. Bring to a boil quickly, then reduce the heat to low, or place the pot on top of a woodstove to replace some humidity.

3. As you enjoy the steam and fragrance, keep a watch on the water level.

4. The potpourri mix will keep in the jar at room temperature indefinitely.

TIP Placing the potpourri in muslin bags or heat-sealable tea bags in advance makes for an easier cleanup.

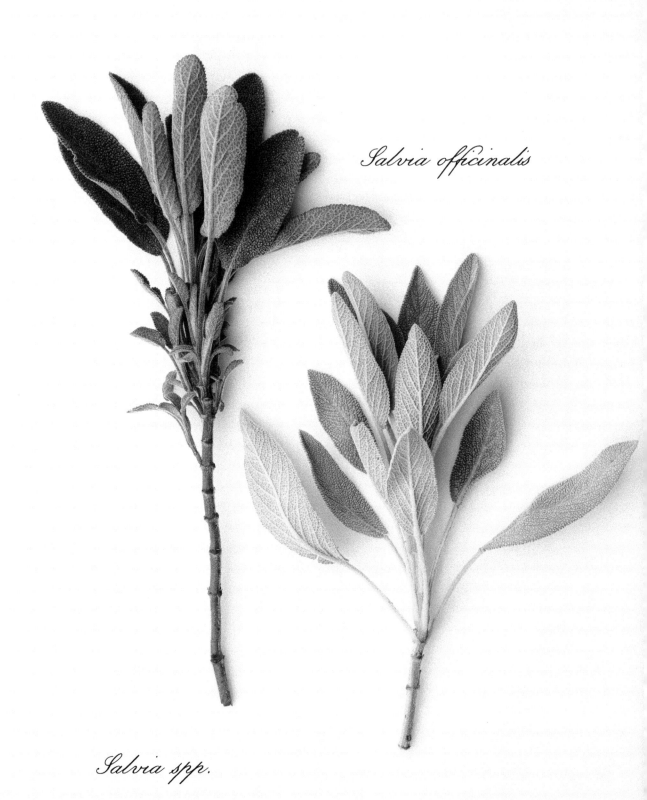

Salvia officinalis

Salvia spp.

SAGE

Sage and rosemary are considered to be "sister herbs" because they share many similar properties. Many of sage's health benefits are derived from the rosmarinic acid prevalent in rosemary, and the two plants are native to the Mediterranean region and grow in similar conditions. Sage's genus name, *Salvia*, derives from the Latin *salvere*, meaning "to be saved" or "salvation." It's a common ritual to burn sage to clear the air of negativity, and as it turns out, sage smoke is truly antibacterial and antimicrobial, keeping all sorts of infections at bay. There are many stunning varieties of sage, each with slightly varied benefits. For instance, *S. bergarten* has large leaves, *S. extrakta* has very high amounts of essential oil, and *S. sclarea* isn't culinary but is highly valued for its antidepressant properties. A sage holds great wisdom, and so it is with the plant.

ABOUT SAGE

OTHER COMMON NAMES common sage, desert sage, garden sage, golden sage, kitchen sage, true sage, culinary sage, Dalmatian sage, tricolor sage, purple sage, clary sage, smudge, broad-leaf sage

SAFETY CONSIDERATIONS Sage essential oil contains thujone, which is possibly a neurotoxin. Do not ingest the essential oil, which is at least 100 times more concentrated than a cup of tea or a teaspoon of tincture. Sage is generally recognized to be safe as a food, and in quantities typically used as food. Avoid excessive, prolonged use, particularly if you are pregnant or have a seizure disorder or diabetes.

PART USED leaf

ENERGETICS warm, dry, slightly bitter

PROPERTIES Sage is antibacterial, antifungal, anti-inflammatory, antiseptic, antispasmodic, astringent, antiviral, and carminative. It may also alleviate rheumatoid arthritis.

USES One of the highest virtues of sage is its ability to dry and tone dampness. Externally, this means policing those folds and creases where fungus likes to hang out and drying up excess oils, excretions, and weepy skin conditions. Internally, sage goes after excess mucus, firms up membranes, and can help with excessive perspiration or saliva. Sage also helps mothers dry up their milk when weaning children off breastfeeding. Sage leaves are usually long ovals, thick, strong, and pebbly, like a tongue. It makes sense, then, that it helps with mouth, gum, and throat issues. It is calming and grounding when used either internally or topically. It has been used traditionally to bring down fevers and promote sleep. Menopausal hot flashes respond well to sage tea or tincture. Sage has been found to be capable of killing *E. coli*, and there's a good chance that the essential oils of sage and various other aromatic herbs will be what saves us from MRSA in the next decade or so. Sage tea with meals promotes digestion and helps with stomach pain, excess gas, diarrhea, bloating, and heartburn.

PREPARATIONS teas, tinctures, vinegars, capsules, skin creams, lotions, and soaps

DOSAGE It's safe to ingest three to four cups of tea or droppers of tincture a day. Follow directions on capsules. Sage is safe for topical use as needed.

GROWING TIP Sage is very easy to grow. Check with your garden nursery for hardiness information in your region. Sage needs good drainage, good air circulation, and plenty of sunshine. Even in the middle of a cold winter I can usually find some usable leaves.

Home treatments

The teen years (and menopausal years, now that I think about it) are fraught with sweaty palms, oily hair and face, and just too much dampness all around. Make a sage facial by grinding sage together with oatmeal, yarrow, and roses to take away the oil slick. Sage tea can help with excessive perspiration.

For a brutal sore throat or laryngitis, sage tea is a wonder. When it was first suggested to me, I recall being confused—it seemed like drying out my throat would only make things worse. But I found that it toned the soft tissue of my palate and throat, handily took care of the inflammation, and cleared the mucus away.

SAGE AND GARLIC SOUP

Makes about 8 cups
Prep time: 45 minutes

This is a great nourishing soup to have for a wet, drippy head cold, or heavily productive respiratory infection. The garlic comes out to do the heavy lifting, and the sage backs it up all the way.

INGREDIENTS

1 head garlic, cloves peeled and minced or crushed

½ cup fresh sage leaves, coarsely chopped

¼ cup fresh thyme leaves

¼ cup fresh parsley, coarsely chopped

2 teaspoons minced fresh gingerroot

1 pinch cayenne

6 cups chicken or vegetable broth

6 large egg yolks, beaten

Salt and freshly ground black pepper

SUPPLIES

a large pot

1. In a large pot, combine all the ingredients except for the egg yolks, and bring to a boil over high heat.

2. Reduce the heat to low and simmer, uncovered, for 25 minutes.

3. Add a splash of hot soup to the egg yolks. While whisking, slowly pour the yolk mixture into the soup.

4. Season with salt and pepper.

TIP Eat this soup a couple of times a day, and you'll be back to normal in no time.

SAGE AND LEMON HONEY

Makes 8 to 10 ounces
Prep time: 30 minutes

In this delicious concoction, the lemon and honey gradually meld into a light syrup, punctuated by the sage. It's tasty and good medicine. If you're an adventurous cook, try it in some dishes as well.

INGREDIENTS

2 lemons, thinly sliced with seeds removed

½ cup fresh sage leaves, finely chopped

6 to 8 ounces raw local honey

SUPPLIES

a 1-pint jar

a skewer

1. Combine the lemon slices and sage leaves in a pint jar.

2. Pour the honey over the lemon and sage, completely covering them.

3. Poke around the mixture with a skewer to get all the air bubbles out.

4. Cover and refrigerate. The honey will keep for up to 1 year.

TIP Use by the spoonful in healing teas.

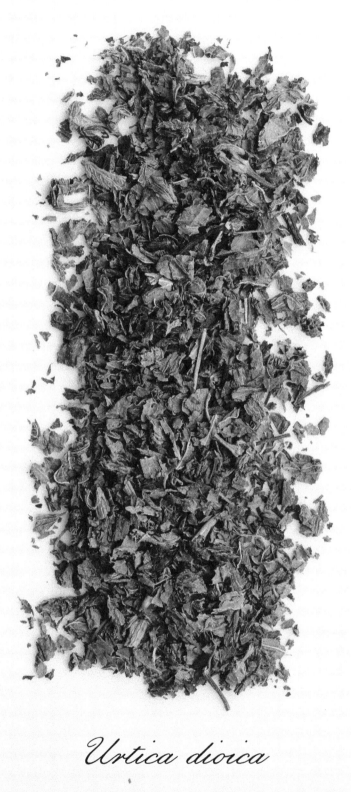

Urtica dioica

STINGING NETTLE

Most country kids remember stinging nettle about as unhappily as they
remember electrical fences. It grew in the
cow pasture I had to cross to get to the
stream where we spent long summer days.
Barefoot, in shorts and sleeveless shirts, I
got to know that sting pretty well. I didn't
know about all of stinging nettle's benefits, though. The Latin name comes from
uro, meaning "to burn." The underside of
the leaves and the stems are covered with
small, hollow, needle-like, stinging hairs,
called trichomes, which deliver an injection
of histamine that cause redness, welts,
and a mighty sting.

In addition to all of its medicinal
properties, nettle has become one of my
favorite vegetables. I even planted a patch
next to the house so that I could have it
often. For food or medicine, nettle must
be used prior to blooming, so I keep mine
mowed for new growth.

ABOUT STINGING NETTLE

OTHER COMMON NAMES nettles, burn hazel

SAFETY CONSIDERATIONS Those taking blood-thinning, blood pressure, or diuretic medications should avoid nettles, as they may amplify the effects of the pharmaceuticals.

PARTS USED leaves, roots

ENERGETICS dry, hot, sweet, salty

PROPERTIES Nettle is antibacterial, anti-inflammatory, astringent, antihistamine, decongestive, diuretic, expectorant, galactagogue, nutritive, styptic, and tonic. It is possibly one of the best plant sources of bioavailable vitamins and minerals out there, full of vitamin A, various B vitamins, vitamin C, amino acids, boron, calcium, copper, fatty acids, folic acid, iron, magnesium, manganese, phosphorus, potassium, and zinc.

USES Being astringent and antibacterial, nettle soothes eczema while fighting allergic responses. It is a good source of iron, and the vitamin C content increases absorption. A mixture of nettle root and saw palmetto berry shows promise for helping men over age 50 who have difficulty with the lower urinary tract due to benign prostatic hyperplasia. Nettle is a treasured woman's herb from cradle to grave. Nettles even out hormones and alleviate PMS symptoms, help with excessive bleeding, support the nursing mother with milk production, and, finally, guide us through and beyond menopause by supporting the adrenals and the endocrine system.

Some believe that the stings interfere with the way the body transmits pain signals by temporarily wearing out the "transmitter" so that pain signals aren't received. The sting is sometimes intentionally administered in a process called urtification on painful joints caused by osteoarthritis or rheumatoid arthritis. The tea is effective as a pain reliever, and can be used in combination with an external application.

PREPARATIONS tinctures, teas, nourishing herbal infusion, creams and salves, pills or capsules, vinegars, and hair care products

DOSAGE For tincture, tea, or vinegar, daily use up to four times a day is fine. Follow label directions for commercial capsules. Homemade pills can be taken several times a day. Nettle is safe to use externally as needed.

GROWING TIP I planted one small nettle plant three years ago. It is now a 6-foot round plot, growing by the day. I strongly suggest using raised beds or sinking a metal barrier into the soil to contain nettles.

Home treatments

In the dead of winter where I live, there are always allergens in the air, and my kids have serious allergies. We've tried many things over the years, finally settling on a combination of stinging nettles and bee pollen, which has proven to be about 85 percent effective! We take a teaspoon of bee pollen throughout the day along with a nettle tincture or tea three times a day.

During the beginning stages of menopause, menses can become heavy and more frequent, sometimes leading to anemia. Time for nettle to shine! Daily doses of a highly concentrated herbal infusion (mix 1 ounce of dried herb with 1 quart of heated water and steep overnight) can help balance out the confused hormones and rebuild iron.

BLACK NETTLE SYRUP

Makes about 4 cups
*Prep time: 45 minutes, plus 2 to 3
hours to steep*

This recipe is credited to Adrian
White of Deer Nation Herbs.
Fortifying the nettles with mineral-
rich blackstrap molasses is a stroke
of genius. I think blackstrap molasses
tastes like brown sugar, and I have
no trouble taking the syrup straight.
If the taste or smell of this syrup is
objectionable to you (the mere mention made my mother shudder), mix
it with cereal or hot tea, or bake some
molasses cookies.

INGREDIENTS

3 cups water

1 cup dried stinging nettles

2 cups organic honey

12 ounces blackstrap molasses

SUPPLIES

2 small saucepans

1 tinted glass jar or other container

1. In a small saucepan over low
   heat, combine the water and
   nettles. Gently simmer for 10 to
   15 minutes. Cover and either
   remove from the heat or keep
   over low heat and let steep for
   2 to 3 hours.

2. Strain the syrup and transfer to a
   clean saucepan.

3. Add the honey and bring up to a
   simmer again over low heat, until
   the mixture reaches a consistency
   you like. I usually reduce by about
   a third.

4. Add the molasses to the mixture
   and stir while hot. Let cool.

5. Transfer the cooled syrup to your
   desired container, preferably an
   amber-tinted glass jar. Store the
   syrup in the refrigerator and use
   within a year.

STEAMED NETTLES

Makes about 1 cup
Prep time: 5 minutes, plus 30 minutes to pick the nettles

Steaming nettles briefly, even for a minute, causes the trichomes to break, rendering them stingless. There is something about the flavor of steamed fresh nettles that is deeply nourishing. To me, they taste as if they can make one whole again.

INGREDIENTS

4 cups fresh stinging nettles

½ cup water

½ tablespoon butter

Salt

SUPPLIES

gloves

a small saucepan

1. Using gloves, pinch the tops from the nettle plants.

2. Toss into a colander and rinse.

3. In small saucepan, bring the water to a boil.

4. Add the nettles, cover, and steam for about 3 minutes.

5. Drain, then return to the saucepan. Stir in the butter, season with salt, and serve.

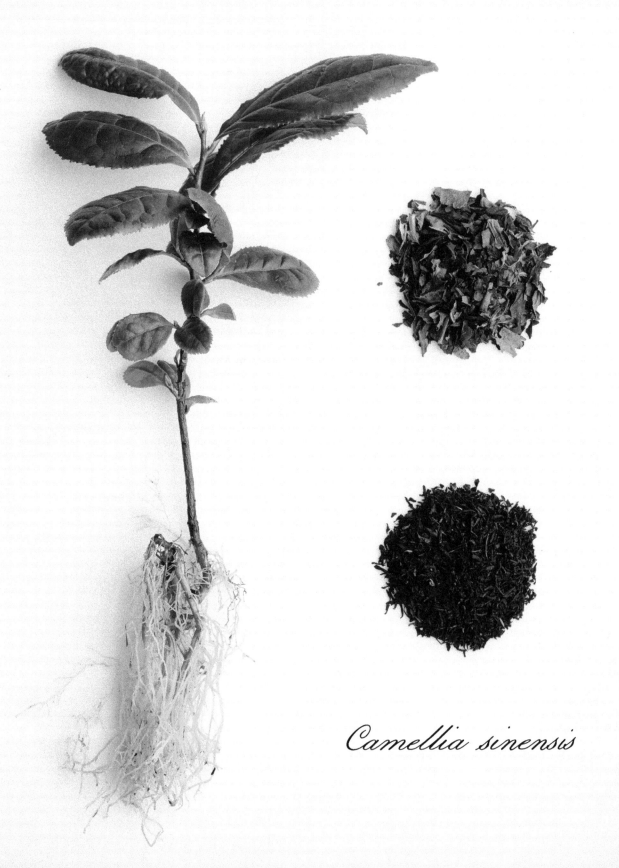

Camellia sinensis

TEA

We rarely talk about all of the health benefits of tea, or the tea plant, but it is full of herbal goodness. The same plant that fills the boxes of tea bags in the grocery store aisle is responsible for black tea, green tea, oolong tea, white tea, kukicha (twig), pu'er, matcha, yellow tea, and dark tea. They are processed or harvested differently to obtain a particular type of finished tea. Elements such as elevation, median temperature, and soil condition determine the quality of teas. Tea is one of the most popular beverages in the world; it is part of ceremonies and rituals, and even has its own class of experts, called tea sommeliers. The U.S. currently lags behind the rest of the world in tea consumption, but it is quickly catching up.

ABOUT TEA

OTHER COMMON NAMES chai, Ceylon tea, green tip, dragon pearls, orange pekoe

SAFETY CONSIDERATIONS Tea contains caffeine, so those sensitive to that should avoid it.

PARTS USED leaves and twigs

ENERGETIC cool, dry, astringent, sweet, bitter

PROPERTIES Tea is antibacterial, antioxidant, immune-stimulating, and anti-stress.

USES Green or white tea may be helpful in maintaining a healthy weight, and many miracle claims have been made to that effect. But if there were miracle herbs, there would be no overweight herbalists, so always keep that in mind. The presence of antioxidants in tea is well known. Tea is one of the only three known sources of L-theanine, an amino acid that improves sleep and is calming, relaxing, and stress- and anxiety-reducing. All teas made from *Camellia sinensis* have catechins, a type of polyphenol that is thought to fight disease and stimulate the metabolism. EGCG (epigallocatechin gallate), thought to be one of the most important catechins, is prominent in green tea. To increase bioavailability of the catechins, add lots of freshly squeezed lemon juice. The popular commercial beverage that is half lemonade and half tea is about perfect when made at home with real lemon, green tea, and fresh stevia leaves.

PREPARATIONS Teas are available loose, packaged in tea bags, powdered (in the case of matcha), as green tea capsules, infusions, and compresses, and used in cooking.

DOSAGE Tea is generally considered safe, although keep in mind that it contains caffeine. Five cups per day is suggested for getting an optimal amount of EGCG from green tea.

DRINKING TIP Bagged tea is okay, but it is to tea what dried herbs in tins are to homegrown fresh herbs. We owe it to ourselves to use loose teas and taste the difference. Most tea bags are filled with "tailings," the small powdered bits that are left after the good stuff has been packaged as loose tea.

Home treatments

Sitting down to write about tea, something struck me. Over the last year, I've been working on getting into better shape and, coincidentally, have been regularly drinking green tea. A couple of months ago I stopped and switched to water. I have otherwise done everything the same but have lost no more weight. You know what I'm going to brew up tonight! In any case, I have found the beverage to be calming and energizing at the same time. Not sweating the small stuff frees up a lot of energy to do things that are more enjoyable.

Tea is very good for oral health. Swap in some stevia for sugar or honey, and tea may lower bacteria in the mouth, protecting against cavities, gum disease, and even bad breath. The astringent properties can help with sores, and if you're like me and bite your cheeks, it also helps settle that down so the area doesn't get bitten again and again.

BUTTER TEA

Makes about 4 cups
Prep time: 15 minutes

Butter tea is a traditional beverage from Tibet that we might consider more of a mild broth than a tea. The main taste is salt, with the tea and dairy closely following. Some say it is an acquired taste, but I've come to love this warming and comforting brew. It is worth getting to know.

INGREDIENTS

4 cups water

3 teaspoons dried black tea leaves or similarly sized chunk of pressed tea

¼ teaspoon salt

2 tablespoons butter

⅓ cup full-fat goat milk (unless you have access to the traditional yak milk, that is)

SUPPLIES

a saucepan

a blender

1. In a saucepan, bring the water to a boil.

2. Add the tea leaves, reduce the heat to low, and simmer for at least 5 minutes.

3. Strain and return the liquid to the pot.

4. Add the salt, butter, and milk.

5. Pour the liquid into a blender and blend for 3 or 4 minutes.

6. Serve immediately.

MATCHA AND GINGER ELECTUARY

Makes about 4 ounces (10 to 12 servings)
Prep time: 15 minutes

For this recipe, you can substitute any type of tea for the matcha, as long as the tea is finely ground. To mix up the flavor, try adding other ingredients like cinnamon, lemon, or finely ground dried berries. The ginger adds a little zip.

INGREDIENTS

2½ tablespoons matcha powder

1 heaping teaspoon powdered ginger

3 ounces honey

SUPPLIES

a jar

1. In a bowl, mix together the matcha powder, ginger, and honey to form a paste, adjusting the ingredients as necessary to reach the consistency you'd prefer. If the mixture is too dry, add more honey; if it's too runny, add more matcha.

2. Transfer the electuary to a jar.

3. For a cup of tea, use about a teaspoon of the mixture in hot water, stirring well to dissolve. You can also eat the electuary straight from the jar.

4. If the paste is stiff enough, you can dry it and form it into properly sized portions, making this the perfect instant tea mix.

5. The electuary can be stored at room temperature for up to a year.

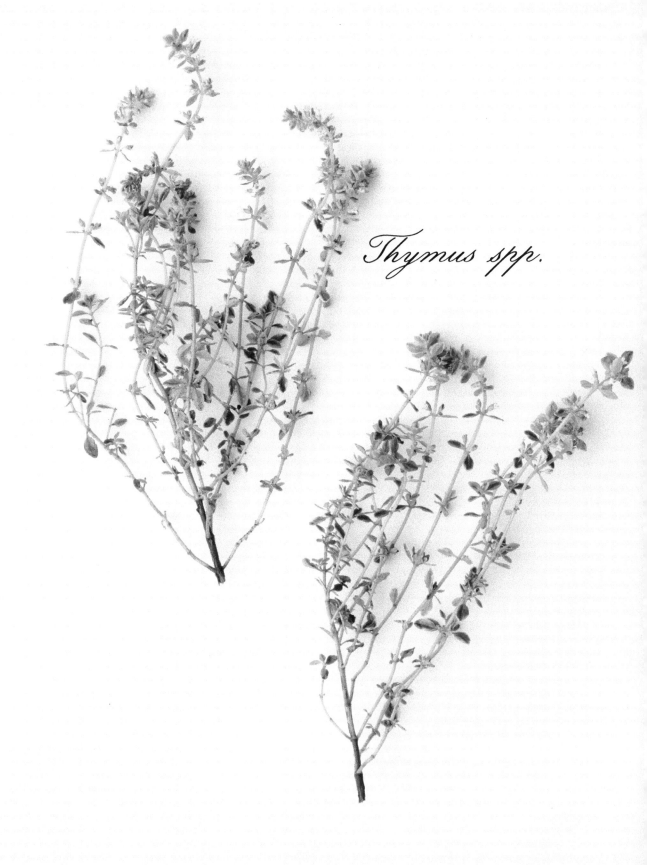

Thymus spp.

THYME

When I was first starting out with culinary herbs, someone told me that thyme was the easiest and most versatile of the savory herbs. I have to agree. In fact, it got to the point where I'd step out and gather a few sprigs to add to almost every dish. Thyme is another Mediterranean herb, like sage and rosemary, and it loves the sun and well-drained soil. This tiny-leafed plant that is only a few inches from the ground has a rich history. It was considered a symbol of courage in medieval times, and later had the honor of being an ingredient in the vinegar known as Four Thieves (or perhaps Forthave's after a doctor of the time) that was used as a preventive for the Black Plague. As if that weren't enough for this diminutive ground cover, it is also a favorite of the fairies.

ABOUT THYME

OTHER COMMON NAMES garden thyme, mother of thyme, wild thyme, creeping thyme, mountain thyme

SAFETY CONSIDERATIONS Thyme contains thymol, so large quantities (generally referring to the use of essential oil) used over an extended period may cause damage to the heart, lungs, kidneys, liver, and nervous system. Never take thyme essential oil internally or use it undiluted on the skin.

PARTS USED leaves and sprigs

ENERGETICS warming, dry, spicy

PROPERTIES The actions of thyme are mostly due to the component thymol in the essential oil, which is present throughout the leaves. It is anodyne, antifungal, antibacterial, antimicrobial, antioxidant, antiseptic, antispasmodic, antiviral, carminative, diaphoretic, expectorant, sedative, and tonic, and is a natural disinfectant. Thyme is a rich source of minerals and vitamins, including vitamin K, which is essential for proper blood clotting. Thyme also contains DHA, an omega-3 fatty acid crucial to brain function.

USES Thyme's antiseptic properties were useful in field hospitals during World War I, saving the lives of many wounded soldiers. Today it is still very valuable in compresses, salves, or washes for acne, scalp problems, rashes, bites, wounds, or parasites, such as scabies and lice. As an antifungal, thyme offers relief from athlete's foot or jock itch. Syrup or tea made from thyme will break up and move excess mucus in chest colds or stuffy heads, while putting the brakes on viral infections. Thyme can help calm coughs and bronchitis, and soothe sore throats while encouraging restful sleep. Like so many aromatic culinary herbs, thyme is great for the digestive tract, improving appetite, relieving excess gas, and improving the absorption of nutrition. As a tea during PMS, the diuretic, anti-inflammatory, and antispasmodic properties are marvelous and carry through during the menses to relieve cramps, pain, and insomnia.

PREPARATIONS teas, tinctures, salves, poultices, essential oils

DOSAGE Use thyme as needed in all preparations, but use extra caution with the essential oil.

HARVESTING TIP It's much easier to separate the leaves from the stems while the thyme plant is fresh. Hold the top of a sprig with one hand, and run the other hand down the length of the stem, stripping it. If you wait until it is dry, the stems often break and fall into the mix.

Home treatments

Thyme is good for any kind of skin issue, from acne, eczema, inflammation, and signs of aging to cuts, wounds, rashes, and bug bites. Thyme's antioxidant, antibacterial, and antiseptic properties make thyme-infused oil, vinegar, or water fantastic for skin health. Purchase a bottle of rubbing alcohol and pour about a cup out. Fill with thyme. After it has infused, put it into a spray bottle and use as an effective skin soother.

In upper-respiratory infections, thyme comes to the fore. Hot tea in a wide mug allows you to drink thyme infusion and inhale the steam. It loosens and gets rid of excess mucus and calms cough spasms. Thyme can induce perspiration and urination, clearing out illness. Thyme is remarkable in its ability to relieve inflammation and pain, resulting in the ability to relax and get to sleep.

FOUR THIEVES VINEGAR

Makes about 1 quart
*Prep time: 15 minutes, plus about 2
weeks to steep*

There are many variations to this
vinegar, so feel free to improvise. All
of these ingredients have spectacular
healing properties. You can use the
vinegar by the spoonful in a glass of
water, or as an ingredient in a meal.

INGREDIENTS

2 tablespoons dried thyme

2 tablespoons dried rosemary

2 tablespoons dried sage

2 tablespoons dried lavender

2 tablespoons dried peppermint

2 tablespoons chopped fresh garlic

1 quart organic raw apple cider vinegar

SUPPLIES

a 1-quart glass jar

1. In a clean 1-quart glass jar,
   combine the herbs and apple
   cider vinegar. Cover and let steep
   in a cool, dark place for about
   2 weeks, shaking daily.

2. When the steeping is finished,
   strain and return the vinegar to
   the jar. Store at room temperature for 6 months.

THYME AND ELDERBERRY COUGH DROPS

Makes 100 to 300 drops, depending on size of the candy
Prep time: about 1 hour

You can make these terrific cough soothers with any herb that calms coughs and scratchy throats.

INGREDIENTS

1 cup strong thyme-elderberry infusion (see page 19)

3 cups sugar

2 tablespoons butter

Confectioners' sugar

SUPPLIES

a large saucepan

a candy thermometer

a glass baking dish

kitchen shears

1. In a large, heavy saucepan off of heat, combine the thyme-elderberry infusion, granulated sugar, and butter, stirring to dissolve the sugar. Turn the heat to medium-high. If cooked too fast, the mixture will try to climb out of the pan and scorch. Boil the mixture until it reaches 300°F on a candy thermometer.

2. Butter a large glass baking dish. When the mixture gets to 300°F, remove from the heat, stir for a minute, and pour it into the baking dish.

3. Sprinkle a table surface or cookie sheet with confectioners' sugar.

4. As the mixture cools, pull up the end of the candy with a fork. Using kitchen shears, cut the candy into pieces and toss into the confectioners' sugar, where it will finish hardening. You can put it in a warm oven (180°F to 200°F, "warm" setting) if the candy is setting up too fast. When the candy sets up, it is hard.

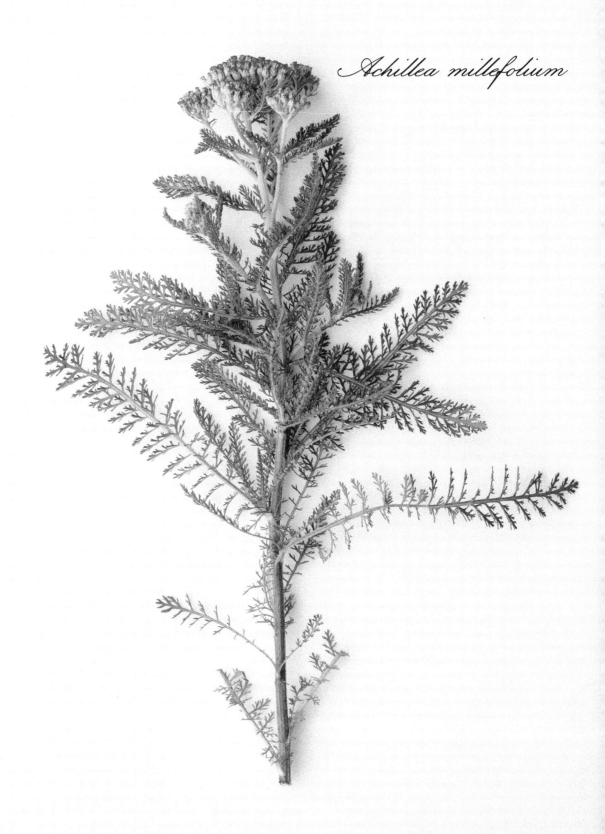

Achillea millefolium

YARROW

Wild yarrow is a common weed in my area. It snuggles up to the bayberry and hazelnut bushes along the path down to the soap workshop, and in early summer I gather the flowers on the way home. To the untrained eye, yarrow might look like Queen Anne's lace, but there are many differences, one being that yarrow's leaves look like green millipedes. The plant is so common, yet I ignored yarrow for a long time. After Ceara Foley from the Appalachia School of Holistic Herbalism talked about how much she loved yarrow at a conference I attended, I researched it deeper. The next spring I was using it in every preparation I could think to make. Now yarrow is one of my go-to herbs.

ABOUT YARROW

OTHER COMMON NAMES woundwort, knight's milfoil, milfoil, nosebleed, devil's nettle, old man's pepper, devil's plaything, bad man's plaything, yarroway, thousand-leaf, soldier's woundwort, bloodwort, carpenter's weed, death flower, staunchweed, field hoop (among many others)

SAFETY CONSIDERATIONS Individuals with clotting disorders should use caution with internal use of yarrow. Avoid yarrow in pregnancy. Fresh yarrow plant may (in rare cases) cause dermatitis, and some people are allergic to yarrow.

PARTS USED all aerial parts

ENERGETICS warm, dry, bitter

PROPERTIES Yarrow is anodyne, astringent, antianxiety, antispasmodic, carminative, diaphoretic, diuretic, febrifugal, anti-inflammatory, relaxing, and styptic, and it tones tissue.

USES Yarrow eases anxiety and stress, and helps relieve insomnia. It also relieves pain and many stomach problems, including nausea, vomiting, gas, bloating, cramps, and diarrhea. The astringency of yarrow makes it brilliant at tightening and healing sore or bleeding gums and toning mucus membranes. As a styptic, yarrow stops bleeding very quickly. Stuffed up a gushing nosebleed, packed into a wound, or wrapped around a wound on the way to the hospital, yarrow can be a lifesaver. Women have long used yarrow internally for heavy bleeding due to uterine fibroids, endometriosis, ovarian cysts, or very heavy periods. Conversely, yarrow can also be used to stimulate menstruation and relieve menopausal night sweats and difficulty sleeping. Yarrow is useful in reducing fevers by encouraging a sweat. It assists in fighting bacteria and infections, acts as a decongestant to ease coughs and sinus infections, and is anti-inflammatory. Yarrow is helpful for seasonal allergies and soothes hives and skin rashes.

PREPARATIONS teas, tinctures, poultices, salves, sitz baths, and bathing herbs

DOSAGE Take tea or tincture three times a day when needed. Externally, you can use a poultice or salve as needed.

TEA TIP Here are a few tea blends to try:

- Blend with echinacea, elderflower, ginger, and peppermint for colds, fevers, and flu-like symptoms.

- Blend with goldenrod and stinging nettle for seasonal allergies.

- Blend with chamomile, linden, and catnip for a restful sleep.

Home treatments

Yarrow's styptic abilities are very important for people who are outdoors working or playing hard. Children should be taught about yarrow and plantain, and older people who may use blood thinners will benefit from the knowledge of yarrow as well. The whole dried herb is uncomfortable and possibly damaging to wounded tissue, but yarrow powder is simple and effective to use.

Yarrow isn't typically the first herb we reach for to relieve stomach problems, but it is a warming bitter after all. If you are overly dry in constitution, don't use yarrow with regularity, but used occasionally for digestive issues, yarrow makes a big difference. Yarrow tea, tincture, or bitters tone the system, trigger various critical digestive actions, and address almost every sort of digestive complaint.

YARROW AND CHAMOMILE BITTERS

Makes about 8 to 10 ounces
Prep time: 15 minutes, plus 1 month
to steep

Bitter tastes have all but disappeared from most of our diets, but we need them for proper digestion. Bitterness signals to the entire digestive tract that food is coming. It immediately triggers salivation, and all along the digestive route, preparations are made to efficiently process the fuel and move it out.

INGREDIENTS

¼ cup dried yarrow

¼ cup dried chamomile

2 tablespoons fennel seeds

2 tablespoons cardamom pods

2 tablespoons licorice root

10 ounces 100-proof vodka

SUPPLIES

a mortar and pestle or coffee grinder

1-pint jar

1. Combine the yarrow, chamomile, fennel seeds, cardamom pods, and licorice root in a mortar and pestle or coffee grinder, and crush but do not powder them. Just break them to release their flavors.

2. Transfer the mixture to a 1-pint jar and cover with the vodka. Seal the jar and let steep for 1 month.

3. Strain and use by the scant dropper before meals to promote healthy digestion.

HEALING HERBAL TUB TEA

Makes about 6 cups
Prep time: 15 minutes

All of the herbs included in this tea are soothing, healing, and terrific for achy, itchy skin or internal discomfort. Soak in the bath for at least 15 minutes. If a fever is present, keep the water tepid.

INGREDIENTS

1 cup yarrow

1 cup lavender

1 cup plantain

1 cup calendula

1 cup rose

1 cup comfrey

SUPPLIES

1 large jar or gallon-size plastic bag

1. Combine all the ingredients in a jar or gallon-size plastic bag and mix well.

2. To use, scoop out about ½ cup of the mixture and put it into a large muslin bag or tie tightly into a washcloth.

3. Put the bag in a large pitcher and fill with very hot water. Let steep for 10 to 15 minutes while you prepare the bath. Pour the infused liquid into the tub, swish, and climb in.

TIP Although this tub tea is wonderful for the whole body, it can be used as a sitz bath for any of the uterine or menstrual issues mentioned on page 212.

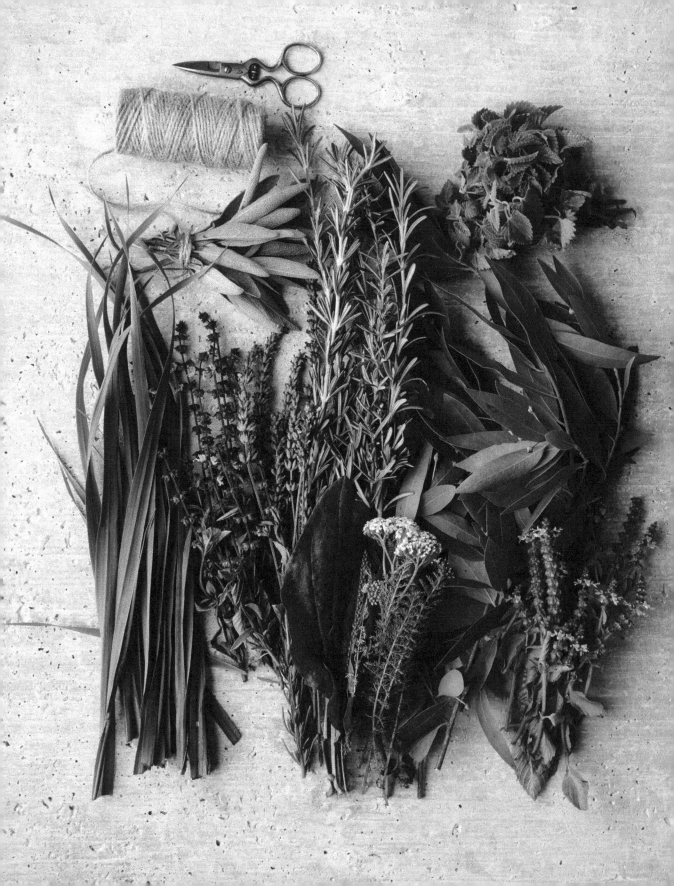

GLOSSARY

ABORTIFACIENT Herbs that are abortifacient can cause a miscarriage and should be avoided in pregnancy.

ACIDIC Having a pH less than 7.

ACRID Sharp or biting in taste or smell. Acrid herbs often "grab" at the back of the throat. A sub-category of *pungent*.

ADAPTOGENS Herbs that help balance, restore, and protect the body.

ADRENAL TONICS Herbs that boost the activity of the adrenal glands while toning and nourishing them.

ALTERATIVE Gradually restores healthy bodily functions.

ANALGESIC Reduces or eliminates pain without causing loss of consciousness.

ANESTHETIC Temporarily depresses neuronal function, producing total or partial loss of sensation.

ANODYNE Soothes or eliminates pain.

ANTIAGING Prevents or lessens the effects of aging.

ANTIARTHRITIC Alleviates or prevents arthritis.

ANTIBACTERIAL Inhibits bacterial growth or kills bacteria.

ANTIBIOTIC Destroys or inhibits the growth of other microorganisms.

ANTI-CATARRHAL Helps remove excess mucus from the body.

ANTICOAGULANT Prevents coagulation of blood.

ANTIDEPRESSANT Treats depression and other conditions.

ANTIFUNGAL Inhibits fungal growth or kills fungi.

ANTIHISTAMINE Blocks the body's histamine reaction.

ANTI-INFLAMMATORY Reduces inflammation in the body.

ANTIMICROBIAL Kills or inhibits the growth of microorganisms.

ANTIOXIDANT Protects cells against the effects of free radicals.

ANTIRHEUMATIC Alleviates or prevents rheumatism.

ANTISEPTIC Prevents infection by inhibiting the growth of microorganisms.

ANTISPASMODIC Relieves spasms in the body.

ANTITUSSIVE Suppresses a cough.

ANTIVIRAL Inhibits viral growth or kills viruses.

APHRODISIAC Elevates, nourishes, and/or sustains intimacy and sensual desire.

AROMATICS Plants with high volatile oil levels that have a strong smell and stimulate the digestive system.

ASTRINGENT Causing shrinkage or constriction of body tissues.

BIOAVAILABILITY The degree and rate at which a substance is absorbed into a living system or is made available at the site of physiological activity.

BITTER Having or being a taste that is sharp, acrid, and unpleasant; not sweet, salty, or sour.

BITTER TONICS Herbs that support the digestive system, boost immunity, and promote overall vitality.

CARMINATIVE Inducing the expulsion of gas from the stomach and intestines.

CATARRH A disorder of inflammation of the mucus membranes in one of the airways or cavities of the body.

CATHARTIC Having purgative action.

COLITIS Inflammation of the colon (large intestine).

DECOCTION A tealike drink produced by boiling herbs in water.

DECONGESTANT Helps relieve nasal congestion in the upper-respiratory tract.

DEMULCENT A usually mucilaginous or oily substance that forms a soothing film over mucus membranes to relieve pain and minor inflammation of that area.

DIAPHORETIC Promotes sweating, helpful for relieving a fever through perspiration.

DISINFECTANT A chemical liquid that destroys bacteria.

DIURETIC Stimulates the flow of urine.

ELIXIR An extract made with herbs, alcohol (generally brandy), and honey.

EMOLLIENT An agent that soothes and protects the skin when applied externally.

EXPECTORANT Promotes and facilitates the discharge of mucus and fluids from the respiratory tract.

FEBRIFUGE A fever-reducing agent.

GALACTAGOGUE Increases the milk supply in a lactating woman.

GRAS (GENERALLY RECOGNIZED AS SAFE) Indicates that consumption of a common kitchen herb in normal food amounts is not likely to cause any serious side effects or adverse reactions.

HEPATIC Acting on the liver.

HYPNOTIC Calming to the point of inducing sleep.

IMMUNE TONICS Herbs that help nourish, tone, and support the immune system.

IMMUNOSTIMULANT An agent that stimulates the immune system. Also known as immune stimulant.

INFUSED OIL An oil, such as olive oil, steeped with dried herbs under low-heat conditions to infuse the oil with the medicinal properties of the herbs. Note: This is not an essential oil.

INFUSION A medicinal remedy made by pouring boiling water over herbs and letting it steep.

LAXATIVE Producing bowel movements.

LINIMENT A topical preparation for application to the skin.

LYMPHATIC Deep-cleans and improves the flow of lymph through the body system.

MARC The solid ingredients (botanicals) that are combined with a liquid to make a tincture.

MENSTRUUM A solvent (alcohol, glycerin, vinegar) used in making tinctures to draw and hold herbal properties.

MUCILAGE A gelatinous substance that contains proteins and polysaccharides and is found in many plants. Herbs that contain mucilage have a slippery texture and mild taste, are soothing and cooling, and are often used topically.

NERVINE Used to calm the nerves.

NEUROPROTECTIVE Serving to protect neurons from injury or degeneration.

NUTRITIVE Serving to nourish the body.

PECTORAL Serving to tonify and strengthen the pulmonary system.

PUNGENT Having a strong taste or smell.

PURGATIVE A strong laxative.

REFRIGERANT A medicine or substance that lowers body heat by cooling the body from the inside out.

RELAXANT A medicine or substance that calms and soothes without being sedating; the act of relaxing contracted tissues.

RESIN A thick, sticky substance that is secreted from a plant.

RESTORATIVE Having the power to restore the body to health.

RUBEFACIENT A topical application that produce redness of the skin, e.g., by causing dilation of the capillaries and an increase in blood circulation.

SEDATIVE Tending to calm, moderate, or tranquilize nervousness or excitement.

SMUDGE A method of burning herbs for purification, ritual, and cleansing.

SPIT POULTICE A simple poultice made by chewing a fresh leaf and applying it directly to a wound.

STIMULANT An agent that energizes a system of the body.

STYPTIC Tending to stop bleeding by constricting tissue and blood vessels.

THERMOGENIC Inducing the production of heat to promote weight loss by increasing the caloric burn rate.

TONICS Herbs that restore or increase body tone.

TRICHOME A hair or hairlike outgrowth on the stems and leaves of plants.

VULNERARY Having wound-healing properties.

Adapted with permission from Kristine Brown, RH (AHG) at Herbal Roots zine (HerbalRootsZine.com).

RESOURCES

First, I encourage you to find a local source for herbs, oils, classes, containers, and supplies. If there is a good shop near you, please patronize them. Find like-minded people in your area. I promise you, they exist. Discussing and experiencing herbs with other people is the very best way to learn. Beyond that, here are some of my favorite resources.

The Essential Herbal Magazine (EssentialHerbal.com) is the print magazine that I edit and publish (it's available in print in the U.S. and as a PDF worldwide). It features articles by people who love herbs and want to share what they know. The magazine covers all aspects of herbs, including medicinal, culinary, crafts, and lore.

Herbal Roots zine (HerbalRootsZine .com) is an amazing online magazine with a focus on teaching children about herbs. It features beautiful artwork and a wide variety of activities, stories, songs, and more, while teaching about one herb each month. It's written and illustrated by Kristine Brown.

American Herbalists Guild (AmericanHerbalistsGuild.com) is an organization of herbalists with listings of schools and registered clinical herbalists. Members are able to take online courses that are given frequently, and there is an annual conference.

United Plant Savers (UnitedPlantSavers .org): Before you head out into the woods with your basket and snippers, learn about the plants that are being overharvested or have lost their habitat. Get information on the ethical harvesting of herbs before you forage.

LearningHerbs and HerbMentor (LearningHerbs.com) is a subscription-based online community featuring a forum, tons of information, interviews with herbalists, and helpful videos. It offers classes frequently and sends out a regular e-newsletter, which typically includes an interesting recipe.

I highly recommend the following books. These women have untold amounts of herbal knowledge and are generous beyond measure in their sharing. If you get a change to attend an in-person lecture with any of them, grab it.

Books

GAIL FAITH EDWARDS (AVAILABLE AT BLESSEDMAINEHERBS.COM)

Herbal Pharmacy: The Art of Herbal Medicine Making
Prayers for the Wild Heart Tribe
Traversing the Wild Terrain of Menopause

ROSEMARY GLADSTAR
(AVAILABLE AT SAGEMOUNTAIN.COM)

Family Herbal: A Guide to Living Life
  With Energy, Health, and Vitality
Herbal Healing for Men
Herbal Healing for Women
Herbal Recipes for Vibrant Health
Herbs for Children's Health
Medicinal Herbs: A Beginner's Guide

SUSAN HESS (COAUTHORED BY ME)

Herbal Medicine Kitchen: The Everyday
Cookbook to Boost Your Health

Herbs and Supplies

BULK APOTHECARY.COM (OHIO)
Bulk apothecary

BULKHERBSTORE.COM (TENNESSEE)
Bulk herb store

IHERB.COM (IOWA)
Frontier retail website for herbs

MOUNTAIN ROSE HERBS.COM (OREGON)
Good-quality organic herbs

SKS-BOTTLE.COM (EAST COAST);
SPECIALTYBOTTLE.COM (WEST COAST)
Bottles, jars, and tins

REMEDY INDEX

AILMENT INDEX

A

Abdominal cramps
  calendula, 49–51
  capsicum, 55–57
  catnip, 61–63
Acne
  dandelion, 79–81
  garlic, 97–99
  ginger, 103–105
  lavender, 127–129
  thyme, 205–207
Adrenal fatigue
  licorice root, 133–135
  oats, 157–159
Allergies, seasonal
  nasturtium, 151–153
  stinging nettle, 193–195
  yarrow, 211–213
Anxiety
  holy basil, 109–111
  hyssop, 121–123
  lavender, 127–129
  linden, 139–141
  oats, 157–159
  tea, 199–201
  yarrow, 211–213
Arthritis pain
  capsicum, 55–57
  catnip, 61–63
  cottonwood, 73–75
  elder, 91–93

  ginger, 103–105
  horseradish, 115–117
  stinging nettle, 193–195
Asthma
  holy basil, 109–111
  hyssop, 121–123
  Mullein, 145–147
Athlete's foot
  cottonwood, 73–75
  nasturtium, 151–153
  thyme, 205–207

B

Blood pressure, high
  capsicum, 55–57
  garlic, 97–99
  rose, 175–177
Blood sugar regulation
  cinnamon, 67–69
  dandelion, 79–81
  garlic, 97–99
Bronchitis
  elder, 91–93
  holy basil, 109–111
  horseradish, 115–117
  licorice root, 133–135
  nasturtium, 151–153
  thyme, 205–207
Burns
  aloe, 37–39
  cottonwood, 73–75

  elder, 91–93
  lavender, 127–129
  plantain, 169–171
  rose, 175–177

C

Cancer
  garlic, 97–99
  rosemary, 181–183
Cholesterol, high
  cinnamon, 67–69
  garlic, 97–99
Circulation
  rose, 175–177
  rosemary, 181–183
Colds and flu
  catnip, 61–63
  echinacea, 85–87
  elder, 91–93
  garlic, 97–99
  holy basil, 109–111
  horseradish, 115–117
  hyssop, 121–123
  nasturtium, 151–153
Colic
  catnip, 61–63
  hyssop, 121–123
Congestion
  horseradish, 115–117
  hyssop, 121–123
  linden, 139–141

nasturtium, 151–153
thyme, 205–207
yarrow, 211–213
Constipation
aloe, 37–39
licorice root, 133–135
plantain, 169–171
Coughs
echinacea, 85–87
garlic, 97–99
horseradish, 115–117
linden, 139–141
Mullein, 145–147
nasturtium, 151–153
thyme, 205–207
yarrow, 211–213
Cradle cap
calendula, 49–51

E

Depression
holy basil, 109–111
oats, 157–159
rosemary, 181–183
Diabetes
capsicum, 55–57
holy basil, 109–111
Diaper rash
calendula, 49–51
cottonwood, 73–75
Digestive issues
aloe, 37–39
calendula, 49–51
capsicum, 55–57
catnip, 61–63
dandelion, 79–81

ginger, 103–105
holy basil, 109–111
horseradish, 115–117
hyssop, 121–123
lavender, 127–129
linden, 139–141
plantain, 169–171
rosemary, 181–183
sage, 187–189
thyme, 205–207
yarrow, 211–213
Dry skin
rose, 175–177

B

Earaches
garlic, 97–99
holy basil, 109–111
Mullein, 145–147
Eczema
aloe, 37–39
cottonwood, 73–75
dandelion, 79–81
holy basil, 109–111
lavender, 127–129
plantain, 169–171
rosemary, 181–183
stinging nettle, 193–195
Edema
dandelion, 79–81

F

Fever
holy basil, 109–111
sage, 187–189

Fibromyalgia
capsicum, 55–57
Fungal infections
cinnamon, 67–69
holy basil, 109–111
lavender, 127–129
nasturtium, 151–153
sage, 187–189
thyme, 205–207

G

Gastrointestinal issues
calendula, 49–51
capsicum, 55–57
cinnamon, 67–69
dandelion, 79–81
lavender, 127–129
licorice root, 133–135
yarrow, 211–213
Gingivitis
aloe, 37–39
tea, 199–201
Gout
dandelion, 79–81
horseradish, 115–117
Grief
linden, 139–141
oats, 157–159

H

Hair and scalp issues
aloe, 37–39
nasturtium, 151–153
rosemary, 181–183
thyme, 205–207

Headaches
  capsicum, 55–57
  catnip, 61–63
  ginger, 103–105
  holy basil, 109–111
  horseradish, 115–117
  lavender, 127–129
  linden, 139–141
  rosemary, 181–183
Heart disease
  capsicum, 55–57
  holy basil, 109–111
Hemorrhoids
  catnip, 61–63
  Mullein, 145–147
  plantain, 169–171
Hives
  catnip, 61–63
  holy basil, 109–111
  yarrow, 211–213
Hyperactivity
  linden, 139–141

I

Illness
  astragalus, 43–45
  Mullein, 145–147
  thyme, 205–207
Infections, skin
  aloe, 37–39
  echinacea, 85–87
  garlic, 97–99
Insect bites and stings
  catnip, 61–63
  cottonwood, 73–75
  echinacea, 85–87

garlic, 97–99
  hyssop, 121–123
  plantain, 169–171
  rose, 175–177
  thyme, 205–207
Insomnia
  catnip, 61–63
  cottonwood, 73–75
  lavender, 127–129
  linden, 139–141
  thyme, 205–207
  yarrow, 211–213
Irritable bowel syndrome
  (IBS)
  aloe, 37–39

J

Joint aches and pains
  capsicum, 55–57
  catnip, 61–63
  cottonwood, 73–75
  echinacea, 85–87
  ginger, 103–105
  horseradish, 115–117
  Mullein, 145–147
  pine, 163–165
  stinging nettle, 193–195

K

Kidney stones
  horseradish, 115–117

M

Memory
  rosemary, 181–183

Menopause
  sage, 187–189
  stinging nettle, 193–195
Menstrual cramps and
  symptoms
  calendula, 49–51
  ginger, 103–105
  lavender, 127–129
  thyme, 205–207
  yarrow, 211–213
Mouth ulcers
  aloe, 37–39
  rose, 175–177
  tea, 199–201
Muscle aches and pains
  capsicum, 55–57
  cottonwood, 73–75
  ginger, 103–105
  horseradish, 115–117
  lavender, 127–129
  Mullein, 145–147
  nasturtium, 151–153
  pine, 163–165

N

Nausea
  cinnamon, 67–69
  ginger, 103–105
  lavender, 127–129
  yarrow, 211–213
Nosebleeds
  yarrow, 211–213

P

Pink eye
  calendula, 49–51

INDEX

ABOUT THE AUTHOR

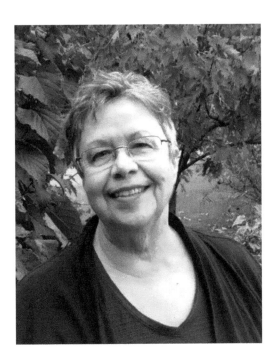

Tina Sams has been enjoying every aspect of plants for nearly her entire life, originally learning from her grandfather in the Pennsylvania German culture of Lancaster, PA. There are few things that are more exciting to her than being elbow deep in herbs, learning about wild edible plants, finding new medicinal uses, or crafting with herbs. Teaming up with her sister Maryanne (the pair have sometimes been known as the Twisted Sisters), she's opened shops, worked festivals, spoken at conferences, taught classes, and run stands at farmers' markets. She is publisher and editor of *The Essential Herbal Magazine*, which she's published for nearly two decades.

CPSIA information can be obtained
at www.ICGtesting.com
Printed in the USA
BVHW020151180919
558750BV00011B/132/P